Creating Change for Complex Children and their Families

of related interest

A Multi-disciplinary Handbook of Child and Adolescent Mental Health for Front-line Professionals
2nd Edition
Nisha Dogra, Andrew Parkin, Fiona Gale and Clay Frake
ISBN 978 1 84310 644 9

The Child's World
The Comprehensive Guide to Assessing Children in Need
2nd Edition
Edited by Jan Horwath
ISBN 978 1 84310 568 8

Making Sense of Child and Family Assessment
How to Interpret Children's Needs
Duncan Helm
Foreword by Brigid Daniel
ISBN 978 1 84310 923 5
Part of the Best Practice in Working with Children series

Children with Complex and Continuing Health Needs
The Experiences of Children, Families and Care Staff
Jaqui Hewitt-Taylor
ISBN 978 1 84310 502 2

Children and Adolescents in Trauma
Creative Therapeutic Approaches
Edited by Chris Nicholson, Michael Irwin and Kedar Nath Dwivedi
Foreword by Peter Wilson
ISBN 978 1 84310 437 7
Part of the Community, Culture and Change series

How to Help Children and Young People with Complex Behavioural Difficulties
A Guide for Practitioners Working in Educational Settings
Ted Cole and Barbara Knowles
Foreword by Joan Pritchard
ISBN 978 1 84905 049 4

Creating Change for Complex Children and their Families

A Multi-Disciplinary Approach to Multi-Family Work

Edited by Jo Holmes, Amelia Oldfield
and Marion Polichroniadis

Foreword by Professor Ian Goodyer

Jessica Kingsley *Publishers*
London and Philadelphia

First published in 2011
by Jessica Kingsley Publishers
116 Pentonville Road
London N1 9JB, UK
and
400 Market Street, Suite 400
Philadelphia, PA 19106, USA

www.jkp.com

Library of Congress Cataloging in Publication Data
Creating change for complex children and their families : a multi-disciplinary approach to multi-family work / edited by Jo Holmes, Amelia Oldfield, and Marion Polichroniadis ; foreword by Ian Goodyer.
    p. ; cm.
Includes bibliographical references and index.
ISBN 978-1-84310-965-5 (alk. paper)
1. Child psychiatry--Case studies. 2. Mentally ill children--Family relationships--Case studies. I. Holmes, Jo. II. Oldfield, Amelia. III. Polichroniadis, Marion.
[DNLM: 1. Mental Disorders--therapy--Case Reports. 2. Child. 3. Family Relations--Case Reports. 4. Social Environment--Case Reports. WS 350.2]
RJ499.C658 2011
618.92'89--dc22
                                    2010052166

British Library Cataloguing in Publication Data
A CIP catalogue record for this book is available from the British Library

ISBN 978 1 84310 965 5

Printed and bound in Great Britain by the MPG Books Group

Contents

Foreword

The early years of human development are some of the most fascinating and revealing in the whole of the life course. In the first two decades an individual child goes through a series of substantial and remarkable changes physically, mentally and socially. Whilst the majority of children accomplish these tasks successfully within a positive and caring environment within their family, their school and their neighbourhood, for some, individual difficulties and environmental hazards constitute substantial risk to wellbeing. Amongst these at risk children are those who develop emotional and behavioural difficulties and disorders that require professional evaluation and may lead to treatment and management, not only for themselves but also for their families.

Child and adolescent mental health services were designed to undertake the treatment and management of the more severely mentally ill young person. A component of that work involves children with particularly difficult and challenging problems who, for a variety of reasons, are unable to respond to treatment in an outpatient and community setting. For such children there is an essential need for day and inpatient services such as the Croft Child and Family Unit in Cambridge. This book is the culmination of over three decades of work carried out at the Croft; although it is edited by current senior clinicians of the service, it bears testimony to all those who have worked with particularly challenging and complex children and their families in an effort to provide them with resilience to carry on with their lives in a successful and adaptive way.

This book is full of how things can and indeed should be done to facilitate change for the better in moderate and severely emotionally and behaviourally disturbed children. The book is beautifully laid out in 11 chapters and takes the reader on a journey from setting the scene of how the unit addresses complex needs through treatments, interventions and learning in easy-to-read chapters. The book holds together by setting each chapter in a client-centred way: individual children and their families are introduced at the beginning of the book and they are used throughout as illustrations of the methods that are being described. These narratives of child and family are fictional based on fact, and provide a key point of contact in the journey from admission to discharge. At the beginning the reader is taken through how the unit's positive and welcoming environment provides the first empathic contact for even the most troubled and worried child and parents. The key importance of therapeutic engagement, structure and containment, and setting up a nurturing environment are discussed in detail in the early phases of the book and are illustrated by vignettes. The Croft demonstrates the core importance of multi-modal work, that is, working with family members and the wider environment when required, and also multi-method work, utilising the important interventions available by taking different perspectives, whether it be through individual, family, multi-family or group work. It outlines the key importance of being able to access learning and of fostering the child's social world, and the intrapsychic importance of understanding the individual.

The authors' experience as a multi-disciplinary team and the Croft's value as a multi-disciplinary unit are self-evident in the balanced and clear descriptions provided for the variety of techniques used by the staff to ensure that the most therapeutic programme can be given in a personalised way to meet the child's and the family's needs.

This is a delightful read and, importantly, a systematic and clear one. The authors are aware of the importance of clinical science and evidence base; there are references pointing readers to more detailed reading on particular topics. Importantly there is an acknowledgement of the need for audit and evaluation of services purporting to provide effective complex treatment for severely challenging behavioural and emotional disorders in children. This book is a must-read for all those interested in and working in the field of child and adolescent mental health, social care, special needs education and related fields, and I recommend it wholeheartedly.

Ian M. Goodyer
Professor of Child and Adolescent Psychiatry
University of Cambridge
March 2011

Acknowledgements

The editors would like to thank all the families and the children who have attended the Croft Child and Family Unit during the last 20 years, for providing the inspiration for this book.

They would also like to thank the team working at the Croft. This book has been a group effort. Without the encouragement, enthusiasm and hard work of the team, this book would not have been possible.

The editorial team would like to say a special thank you to Phyllis Champion for her careful proofreading and her helpful feedback on the content of the book. Her meticulous attention to detail and her impartial perspective have made the book more readable and accessible.

Particular thanks to Professor Ian Goodyer, who has a longstanding relationship with the Croft Unit and who kindly agreed to write the Foreword, despite his numerous other academic commitments.

Jo would like to thank her colleagues in the department who have guided and supported her over the years. A heartfelt thank you for the tolerance and patience of Duncan, Abi, Bethany and Robert, who have coped with a preoccupied wife and mother over many months.

Amelia would like to thank her husband, David, and her children, Daniel, Paul, Laura and Claire, for their support, patience and tolerance and for putting up with a grumpy, tired and increasingly absent-minded wife and mother. A special thank you to Claire for taking the photographs of the artwork and also to Laura for editing those photographs.

Marion would like to thank her husband Panos and son Tony for their computer wizardry and technical know-how along the way, without which she'd still be trying to sort her way through the book. Thanks also go to her daughter Sophie who shares an interest in the content and has encouraged Marion to persevere as a writer, as a suitable occupation in retirement.

Prologue

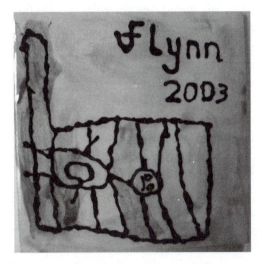

A child who saw the world in a unique way

Background to this book

Working with children with severe and complex mental health needs is both very demanding and rewarding. The editors of this book have worked, for many years, with children (and their families) whose needs are at the severest end of this spectrum. Their experience has been that whilst there are many books written about particular diagnostic groups (e.g. autism spectrum disorder or attention deficit hyperactive disorder (ADHD) or the impact on children of environmental trauma, such as domestic violence or parents who misuse substances) less has been written about the practical approach to working with families with multiple problems. The aim of this book therefore is to share the experience and expertise of the Croft Child and Family Unit with other mental health teams and professionals who support families in other settings, in the hope that there will be both useful ideas and the reassurance of shared dilemmas.

In 2005, the Croft made a video about the unit in collaboration with the media production department at Anglia Ruskin University (Oldfield and Nudds 2005). The aim was to use a visual medium to give children and families an insight into the work of the Croft. Five children were recruited to act the roles of children with psychiatric disorders. Most of the Croft staff were 'themselves' on the video, while a few members of the team acted the roles of the children's parents. The script for the video was written based on cases that had been treated at the Croft in the past, but were sufficiently modified not to be recognisable or to raise issues of confidentiality. The video was very successful, and has been useful to show to families prior to admission as well as when giving talks about the unit to other professionals. The process of making the video enabled the staff team to reflect on the various roles and expertise of specific staff members, as well as to help staff to realise how valuable their own contributions are.

The process of writing this book has been similar. All members of the staff team have contributed. Some have written excerpts or whole chapters, others have spoken about their ideas whilst one of the editors has made notes, and on a couple of occasions day workshops were held where three or four members of the team discussed ideas which were later written up. Once again the process has provoked considerable thought and discussion about the unit's model of care.

Please note that for reasons of convenience we have alternated between using 'he' and 'she' for an unspecified child.

List of contributors
In addition to the three editors, the people who have contributed to this book are as follows:

Nursing team
Mark Careless, Colleen Carpen, Nyssa Cooper, June Everitt, Nina Heaps (lead for Chapter 4), Sandy Hickey, Sharon Kenny (lead for Chapter 3), Andrea King, Andrew Kynaston, Thelma O'Donovan, Kelly Parker, Susan Riley, Lavona Rivington, Phil Ruane, Linda Sammons, Colleen Taylor, Alan Thompson

Medical team
Zeinab Iqbal, Catriona McConnachie

Administrative team
Amanda Lizbinski, Sheran Minton

Domestic team
Geraldine Macfarlane

Teaching team
Anne Harmer, Wendy Nichols (lead for Chapter 6), Susan Parker

Therapists and psychologists
Tina Gutbrod, Vince Hesketh (lead for Chapter 9), Maria Loades, Andrew O'Hahanrahan, Charlotte Wilson (lead for Chapter 8)

External staff support group facilitator
Eleanor Richards

Independent advocate
Sian Williams

Parents (in Chapter 11)
Debbie, Veronica

Children (in Chapter 11)
R, K and T

The families in the book

As in the Croft video made five years earlier (Oldfield and Nudds 2005), it was decided that the families described in this book would be fictional, but would be inspired by the team's past experiences. For reasons of confidentiality, care was taken to ensure that no cases would be too similar to any real clients. A description of each of the fictional children and their families follows. Readers will find out more about each of these families throughout the book, but the following descriptions may be useful for reference.

Arthur

Arthur is six years old. He was referred because he had been excluded from mainstream school after only a few weeks. Various educational settings have been tried, including teaching him on his own with two adults, but he has continued to be highly unpredictable, aggressive and controlling. He will not write or sit at a table. He is very aggressive to other children.

Arthur has one sister who is bright and doing well at school. Both parents are very worried about Arthur – his father, Martin, is a research scientist, who was bullied at school because of a speech impediment. His mother, Angela, used to be a book editor but gave it up to look after the children. She is an orderly and highly organised person. She has a close relationship with her own mother who helps them out a lot but her father was very strict and distant.

At home the difficulties are less marked but Arthur struggles with mealtimes, has poor sleep and frequent temper tantrums.

Arthur has been diagnosed with ADHD and various drugs have been tried. Either they have been ineffective or he has reacted poorly by becoming more aggressive or has lost weight. He has very poor social skills and wants to control social situations. He does not see situations from another's point of view. He has a fascination with maps and road signs. He has marked facial tics.

Although Arthur was initially referred to the Croft for six weeks, some of his difficulties only became apparent in his fifth and sixth week, and it was felt that he and his family would benefit from a longer admission in order to address his complex needs and to help his parents to manage and understand his behaviours.

Philippa

Philippa is 11 years old – she was referred because of severe weight loss over the previous four months. This followed the death of her grandmother, Sue. Her bodyweight is only 65 per cent of that expected for her height. At admission she is only drinking water and eating apples.

Philippa has an older sister, Clare, aged 15, who has severe diabetes. She is well and very bright but has had frequent hospital admissions over the years. They also have a younger sister of five, Anna, who does not appear to have any difficulties.

Philippa's mother, Jane, is quiet and slender. She is a secretary in a building company. She was very close to her own mother and describes herself as very shy as a child. It is not clear if she had any eating problems when she was young. She is a keen marathon runner and Philippa has recently shown an interest in athletics. Philippa's father, Bill, has his own business in digital media. He is at a loss to understand the situation. The parents are wondering if Philippa's eating problem relates to bereavement.

After Philippa's initial eight weeks on the unit her admission was extended by a further four weeks when it was clear that she was making slow but steady progress. It is common for children with severe eating disorders to have longer admissions.

Patrick

Patrick is nine years old. He was referred jointly by the local children and adult mental health (CAMH) service clinic and social services department. His mother, Diane, has mental health problems and his stepfather, Mike, has mobility problems and has been registered disabled for the last ten years.

Patrick has been a lively and challenging child since toddlerhood. His school are very worried about him. He is struggling to learn and he has no stable friendships. He is impulsive and seems to lack any sense of danger. He has recently shown inappropriate sexual behaviour to another child. There are concerns that Patrick may have been sexually abused by one of his mother's previous boyfriends when he was four or five. This man has since been charged with sexual offences against children.

Social services have tried to put in family support but Patrick's behaviour escalates when anyone else is in the family home.

Patrick has a younger sister who also experiences behaviour difficulties at school. There are older half-brothers and sisters from previous relationships who have sporadic contact with the family.

Patrick and his family were offered a six-week admission.

David

David is ten years old and an only child. He is suspected of suffering from post-traumatic stress disorder (PTSD). There are reports that he hears voices, and he has some odd behaviours such as hiding a knife under his bed. He was physically abused by his father who left the household when David was six. David is quiet and able but finds it difficult making friends. He still has occasional contact with his father. They share an interest in football.

David's mother, Sarah, has been severely criminally attacked in the past and has her own emotional difficulties. Before her marriage, she had a successful career in film production and met many well-known celebrities.

David is close to his granny and spends time with her.

David and his mother were offered a six-week admission.

Nick

Nick is 11 years old, and is the last child to arrive on the unit. By the time he arrives, Arthur is in his tenth week, Philippa in her eighth, Patrick in his fifth and David in his fourth. Ben and his mother were admitted the week before Nick arrived. Nick is referred because of severe aggression towards his mother and stepfather. He is excluded from school because of disruptive and antisocial behaviour. He is beginning to get into trouble outside the home, shoplifting with older children, smoking and sometimes drinking. More recently he has started to self-harm, usually after arguments with his mother.

At home he has an intense and conflictual relationship with his mother, Stacey, but is also very anxious about her. Stacey had a very abusive childhood herself and subsequent abusive relationships as an adult. Partnerships are often short-lived. Stacey suffers from depression, and social anxiety. She is isolated, with few friends, and has a difficult relationship with her own mother.

Stacey wonders whether Nick has ADHD and thinks he should be on medication. She feels she has tried everything. She also thinks teachers and other professionals make Nick a scapegoat.

Nick has two younger siblings – they are very wary of him.

Nick and his family have been offered a six-week admission.

Ben

Ben is an 18-month-old toddler referred with his single mother Emma, aged 21.

Emma has been referred by her local CAMH for a six-week parenting capacity assessment.

Emma's history indicates that she has a personality disorder and she appears preoccupied with her own feelings and needs. She is being supported by adult mental health services. Emma has been honest with her health visitor that she is unable to love Ben. She has disclosed that she had been raped as a school-age child and had parents who had their own mental health problems. Social services have been involved in her early years and now Ben is under a child protection plan for neglect. Emma is deemed to be unable to meet Ben's developmental needs, either physically or psychologically. Ben has no structure or routines in his life, and social services have put in a package of care but there has been little change for him. There are accounts of him not being supervised, Emma's drug use is becoming more evident and she is becoming more isolated as she refuses to engage Ben in community activities.

Artwork in the book

All the artwork in the book is by children attending the unit. The tiles were decorated by past Croft children and are currently on display in the waiting area.

Chapter 1

Setting the Scene

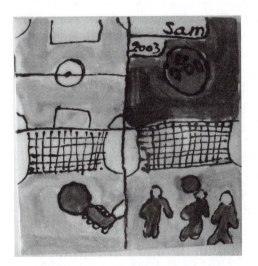

Sam got to know the team through playing football

Patrick is nine. He was referred to the inpatient unit by the local community child mental health clinic and social services department.

Patrick has had longstanding social, emotional and behavioural problems stretching back to toddlerhood. He is very attention seeking and has a wide range of behaviours that cause great concern both to his family and to other adults who come into contact with him. He is becoming increasingly challenging as he gets older. There was a recent incident at school when a younger child reported that Patrick had asked him to show him his willy and to suck his. There are concerns that Patrick may have been sexually abused by one of his mother's previous partners when he was three or four. This man has since been charged with sexual offences against other children.

Patrick's mother Diane has bipolar disorder and has been admitted in crisis to a local mental health hospital a number of times in the past. Patrick's stepfather has chronic back pain and has been registered disabled for the last ten years. He has limited mobility and is low in mood. He has to take high doses of painkillers and this can make him drowsy and lethargic. He lets Patrick's mother take the primary role in Patrick's care.

Diane's mental health is currently reasonably stable. She is taking her medication and attending her appointments with her adult mental health community team. However, she complains of feeling very tired all the time: this is likely to be partly due to her medication. She is also upset about the weight gain from the tablets. She is emotionally warm to Patrick but finds it very hard to put any boundaries around his behaviour. She tends to give in to his demands quickly.

Social services have tried to support the family and Patrick did go to a link family for respite for two weekends but after a confrontation with the father in the link family about his language he jumped out of a window and broke his leg.

At school Patrick has additional adult help in some of his lessons – he has become very attached to one of his helpers but if she is away for any reason his behaviour deteriorates markedly. His relationships with his peers are fragile – he often tries to dominate the group using aggression or antisocial behaviour. Many children in his class are very wary of him. His learning is not progressing well and he has major problems with reading and spelling. His concentration is poor and his mother thinks he may have attention deficit hyperactivity disorder (ADHD). The school are looking for extra resources to provide more one-to-one support for Patrick and think that if they cannot obtain this then his placement at the school may be in jeopardy.

Whilst this is one family's (fictional) story, elements of this scenario will be very familiar to professionals working with vulnerable children and their families. Often professionals are working in situations where there are multiple areas of difficulty and it can be hard to know where to begin. Families may have had extensive contact with a variety of organisations and met many professionals. Their files contain such a mass of paperwork and reports that it is hard for a worker to read them all. Within the documentation there is usually a great deal of evidence of the family's difficulties, but an intervention plan that leads to positive, enduring change is often much more elusive.

So what can be done to help children like Patrick, who, at a very young age, are already showing such serious levels of emotional and behavioural disturbance?

There are many services working with families with complex needs, just like Patrick's family, in a variety of settings. This book has been written by a multi-disciplinary team working intensively with groups of families in a short-term residential health setting. The team describes how they use multi-modal, multi-family approaches to creating the opportunity for change in very vulnerable children and their families. The authors also illustrate the complex relationships that emerge in multi-family work and consider how best to manage these dynamics to achieve the best possible outcome for each family.

The team appreciate that a mental health inpatient unit is an unusual setting for this work and whilst they discuss the unique opportunities that residential work can offer, they also consider how these approaches can be used in other more common community settings.

Children with severe and complex mental health needs

So what is the context for this work? Mental health disorders in children are common: a survey in Great Britain at the turn of the century estimated that 10 per cent of 5- to 15-year-olds have a significant mental health problem (Meltzer *et al.* 2000). This statistic encompassed children with a wide range of disorders ranging from transient anxiety problems related to changes in life circumstances, to children with life-threatening eating disorders or chronic severe mental illness. Research tells us that life outcomes for children struggling with emotional and behavioural disorders are linked to inherent characteristics of the child (e.g. temperament and intelligence), family functioning and community resources. Children living in families that are socially isolated and affected by issues such as domestic violence, substance misuse and parental mental illness are at much greater risk of school failure, unemployment, instability in their own adult relationships and mental health problems in later years.

When considering the group of children with disruptive behaviour disorders, a wide range of therapeutic approaches have been tried, approaches as disparate as psychodynamic play therapy and tranquillising drugs. Research programmes have looked at individual work with children on interpersonal relationships, social skills and anger management. Therapists have also used family therapy treatments and parent support, amongst other methods. Sadly, for the majority of these treatments, there is no clear research evidence of efficacy to support their use.

The exception to this is the use of group parenting programmes such as Webster Stratton, 'The Incredible Years' and 'Triple P' programmes for children with antisocial behaviour (NICE 2006). These programmes place an emphasis on parents developing a positive relationship with their child through praise, rewarding good behaviour and play. They also stress the importance of parents responding consistently and appropriately to antisocial behaviour.

Whilst these programmes can be very useful for parents of difficult children, they are often less successful for parents of older children and adolescents, and there is often a high drop-out rate from the more socially disadvantaged parents – probably the parents who might benefit the most from acquiring these skills.

The existence of this group that is hard to reach was recently highlighted in the review of the Sure Start programme in the UK (Rutter 2006). This was a government initiative aimed at providing additional support to parents of preschool children in the areas of highest social deprivation. Evaluation of this programme showed that whilst significant sections of the population accessed the additional Sure Start resources (such as mother and child play sessions, and funded nursery places), the most vulnerable families often did not.

Sadly, for the most challenging children, with the poorest social support, a tragic outcome is the breakdown of their family relationships, resulting in their placement in alternative care. In Britain such children are referred to as 'looked after children'. Most will be cared for in foster homes, with a small number in residential schools or children's homes. Whilst this alternative care can reduce the risk of immediate harm to a child and provide a safe, containing and, it is hoped, nurturing environment, the process of being removed from the biological family all too often leads to an irreversible breakdown in the child's sense of belonging to that family. Unfortunately, the outcomes for looked after children after they graduate from the care system are very poor (Stein 2004), and most young people face ongoing social problems, unemployment, early parenthood and increased rates of mental health problems.

Intensive family work

Over the last couple of decades there has been increasing recognition that effective interventions with very complex children in multi-problem families require what has been called a multi-modal approach. This approach has been well documented by Dr Scott Henggeler who has described the development and application of multi-systemic therapy (MST) (Henggeler *et al.* 1993, 2009). This is an approach which allocates individual therapists who develop an intense relationship with the members of each family – visiting many times a week and being available 24 hours a day over a period of months. The MST therapist provides advice and practical support to help the families overcome their problems.

This approach has been successfully used with offending adolescents and their families and has been shown to reduce the rate of re-offending behaviour. The motto of MST is 'whatever it takes', and MST workers are trained to work in a holistic way with young people and their parents, tackling education, community inclusion, problematic behaviours, family relationships, and so on. There is an emphasis on a relationship with a single therapist and minimisation of involvement of multiple agencies. Importantly this therapy emphasises the need for therapists to have high levels of support themselves to prevent burnout and to maintain their focus on therapeutic targets.

Multi-family group work

More recently there has been the use of multi-family group work to provide a useful and productive context for families to explore and reflect on their own strengths and difficulties alongside other families experiencing similar problems. Multi-family group work is one of the fundamental approaches used within the Croft Unit and this will be described in depth in Chapter 5. This approach has also been used within dialectical behavioural therapy (DBT) (Linehan, Dimeff and Koerner 2007), a treatment for adults and adolescents with borderline personality disorders. Multi-family group therapy has also shown positive results in eating disorder research programmes.

In addition multi-family group work is a key element of the Mellow Parenting approach designed by Christine Puckering and colleagues in Glasgow (Puckering 2004; Puckering *et al.* 1994), which aims to improve attachment security and emotional warmth between mothers who have been identified as having emotionally abusive relationships with their child. This is described further in Chapter 5.

Residential family treatment

The Croft Child and Family Unit is a 12-bedded unit offering day and inpatient mental health care for children with severe emotional and behavioural difficulties and their families. The unit has been in existence since the 1970s and offers services for children up to the age of 12 or 13; in the UK this covers the primary stage of formal schooling. The unit is part of the British National Health Service (NHS) and is one of only eight such units across the country offering residential mental health care for children. However, the Croft is the only unit in this group that routinely admits children with their parents and treats the family as a whole.

The unit has evolved from a very small day-patient service offering a local service to the children of Cambridge to a residential unit taking referrals from most of the Eastern Region of England – a predominantly rural area with pockets of high levels of deprivation and a population of approximately three million people.

From its inception the unit has always had a high level of contact with parents and a core principle of the service is that children can only be fully assessed and understood within their family group. Commissioners of the service question this principle from time to time as it clearly adds some additional costs to an admission. However, the average admission of a family group to the service is around six weeks, whilst admission lengths in other children's units in the UK are on average twice this length (O'Herlihy et al. 2001). Admitting children with their parents also reduces their stress as they settle into the unit as well as helping us to assess the family as a whole. In addition it gives the opportunity to work with parents and families in multi-group settings.

The unit is part of a mental health organisation that offers care across the lifespan. Most referrals to the service come from NHS teams based in the community – primarily child and adolescent mental health teams and community paediatric teams. Some referrals come from social services teams and from the education system.

Most children and families stay on the unit during the week and return to their own homes at the weekend. On average families spend between six and eight weeks staying at the unit but some may have longer stays.

The team

The multi-disciplinary team consists of nurses, a consultant child and adolescent psychiatrist, a paediatrician, a family therapist, a psychologist, teachers, music therapists, a social worker, a play therapist, a housekeeper and administrative staff.

The children and their families

Children are referred to the unit for a wide range of reasons. Looking back at referral patterns over the last few years, common reasons for referral are:

- assessment and treatment of children with severely challenging behaviour involving risk of harm to themselves or others

- assessment and treatment of children with severe emotional disorder unresponsive to community input

- treatment of children with life-threatening eating disorders

- assessment of children with complex neuro-developmental disorders where diagnostic clarity has not been possible in outpatient settings

- assessment and treatment of children with severely disordered attachment

- re-assessment of children who have chronic difficulties who have been unresponsive to community treatment or whose difficulties are worsening despite maximal outpatient care.

For some children and families there will be multiple areas of concern, but the common theme for all is that the severity of their difficulties has outstripped the resources of community-based services.

In addition to the reasons for referral described above, around ten per cent of our admissions involve a request for a formal assessment of parenting capacity in parents with identified mental health problems. These assessments are discussed in more detail in later chapters.

Summary

This chapter has outlined the context of intensive mental health treatment for pre-pubertal children with complex needs living in complex families. It has introduced some of the models involving parents and multi-family group work that underpins the therapeutic approach used by the inpatient unit described in this book.

Contributors now go on to describe the process of engagement with families and the role of containment and nurturance as a foundation for therapeutic work. Later chapters look at multi-modal approaches to assessment and treatment and the tensions and opportunities that arise in intensive mental health care. Throughout the book there are frequent references to the impact of relationships between families, children and staff, and how these complex dynamics create opportunities for families and staff alike to re-evaluate their belief systems and to try different behaviours.

The final chapter considers how the efficacy of the service can be measured, and contains accounts from children and parents of their experiences during their treatment.

It is hoped that the ideas and experiences explored in this book will be valuable to professionals working in a wide range of settings including residential homes and schools for children with additional needs, paediatric settings, looked after children's care, children's centres, outreach and crisis intervention teams and special education services, to name but a few.

Chapter 2

Therapeutic Engagement

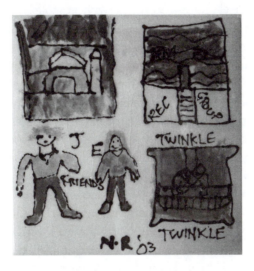

N.R. made friends for the first time

Introduction

With any social encounter, the initial impressions and experience of a first meeting are critical to the success or otherwise of the relationship. Everyone can recall a first meeting that has either drawn them in to a relationship or repelled them. In ordinary circumstances a negative first impression can be repaired if there is an opportunity to give someone another chance and to spend more time with them. But service users, such as Patrick's mother Diane, will have met numerous professionals over the years, some of whom will have been helpful but many of whom she will have met in difficult circumstances. Some professionals may well have needed to say very negative or critical things to her about her care of her children. Naturally she will be anxious and defensive about meeting yet another set of professionals who will ask intrusive questions about her family life and background and who will be making judgements about the way she cares for her children.

So what can be done to make this first phase of engagement as successful as possible?

Be prepared

First, it is important to try to ensure that the team have as much information about a family as possible – to inform them of the issues that are of concern and also to minimise the need for the family to go over their story yet again. Often families will be grappling with very traumatic experiences – bereavement, separation or divorce, abuse – and for a complete stranger to start asking about these issues when they have told their story many times before will both be traumatic in itself and give the family the impression that no thought has been given to them before the meeting.

Whilst obtaining information would seem an obvious need, there are some pitfalls – previous documents may be inaccurate or misleading, and it is all too easy to subconsciously absorb the viewpoint or bias of the author of a report and let this overly influence thinking about a family before even meeting them. These dangers have led some practitioners to advocate commencing a contact with a family without having seen any previous information in order to allow the family to start with a clean slate.

Services offering intensive interventions know that if families decide to engage with them there will be many opportunities to hear their story as the weeks go past – so there is less need to focus on obtaining comprehensive information from the family in the first meeting and more emphasis can be given to establishing the beginning of what one hopes will be a positive relationship.

Information giving

When a family come into contact with one of the helping agencies often there is an information imbalance – the professionals may know a great deal about the family whilst the family may know very little about the service they have been referred to. Evidence shows that the more information people have about the treatment or service they are being offered, the more likely they are to engage.

These days the wonders of modern technology offer many more options than the traditional service leaflet. Like many other services the Croft has developed a website with information aimed at parents, children and professional colleagues (see www. thecroftchildandfamilyunit.nhs.uk). For families with access to the internet this is a valuable resource that gives information about what the unit offers, photographs of members of staff and of the building itself, and a short excerpt from a video. This is often particularly helpful for children (and adults) who are anxious about new environments and it allows them to access information in the safety of their own home. There are also links to other sources of support and advice. Feedback from service users on the website informs its regular editing and re-shaping.

As the leaflets and website were being developed the team was very aware that not all service users can access information through the written word. The music therapist suggested that a video or DVD of the work done at the unit would help families understand more of what is on offer and how the service works, and be particularly helpful to children who are often more engaged by visual media. Months later, with the help of child actors alongside staff members, a 45-minute video was created showing a group of five fictional children going through the programme. This video can be sent to potential service users before their first meeting and feedback from viewers has been good. From time to time, as staff members introduce themselves, family members will say they know who they are already as they have 'seen them on the telly'.

Saying hello and having a cup of tea

The first member of the team that a service user will talk to is usually one of the administrative team. They man the phones and the reception desk and the warmth of their approach to families sets the tone for the whole team. How different is the experience of telephoning a big corporation or government agency and listening to a robotic voice giving you a seemingly endless choice of numbers, from hearing a cheerful human voice saying 'Good morning, how can I help you?'

When families arrive they have frequently endured long, tortuous journeys, with anxious children who might struggle to manage a trip to the local supermarket. Usually the whole family is stressed and ambivalent about the prospect of meeting yet another set of professionals. So to be met with a smile and an offer of a warm drink or glass of juice can help to smooth a difficult moment. As the service offers families a residential stay the team strongly feel that being hospitable, in the same way one would if a visitor called at home, signals to families that they are welcome and that the team is thinking of their comfort before anything else.

Meeting David for the first time

David's family were half an hour late for their first meeting – his mother, Sarah, rang to say that it had been very difficult to get David into the car and she had to ask her brother to come with her to help. David had tried to open the car door on the motorway and they had had to stop and put the child locks on the doors. Later on he had tried to strangle his uncle who was driving so Sarah had to hold his hands for the rest of the journey.

When they arrived at the unit David refused to get out of the car. Sarah came in alone – she was upset and exhausted and very angry with David. The reception team reassured her that often children find it difficult to come in. They made her a drink and the clinicians offered to meet David with her in the car. The next ten minutes was spent trying to engage David in some conversation, to no avail – when the doctor tried to talk to David's mother about her concerns David started kicking the dashboard. Sarah agreed that it was best to carry on the conversation inside the unit and David stayed in the car with his uncle and one of the nurses. After Sarah had gone the nurse talked with his uncle about football. David appeared to be listening and after a few minutes he started to join in with occasional nods and odd comments. A little later the nurse suggested that David might like to kick a ball around in the garden with him.

Half an hour later David said he was thirsty and they went into the unit for a drink and a biscuit. As they walked through the unit the nurse told David a little bit about the sort of activities the children do during the week and David muttered that he loved going swimming. After his biscuit David asked about his mum and he went to find her in one of the playrooms just in time to hear a little more about what happens at the unit.

By this time Sarah had been able to talk about her worries about David without him being present and she admitted that it had been much easier for her to be frank, as she knew that he hated hearing her talking about his problems.

Supporting the 'meeters and greeters'

In any organisation the administrative team is always the key department to keeping the system running smoothly. In an inpatient ward setting administrators have to cope with many tasks – making families welcome, typing letters on time, keeping paperwork in order and staying calm in the face of everyone arriving in reception at the same time and needing their piece of work done immediately. In addition receptionists are often answering the telephone to people in distressed states (both service users and colleagues), and as they sit across the reception desk from the waiting area, they may witness very challenging behaviours and very negative family interactions – sometimes interactions that families would be anxious not to show to mental health professionals. So supporting the administrative team in managing these emotional situations and valuing their observations should not be overlooked. In the Croft team this means frequent communication between clinicians and administrators – seeking their views, asking how they are and valuing them as an important part of the assessment team.

The first meeting

It is all too easy for professionals to forget how it feels for a family to meet a doctor, psychologist or nurse for the first time. Clinicians are so accustomed to meeting new people in a situation where they are in control that they can overlook the uncertainty and anxiety this can evoke, however skilled they may be at putting people at ease.

Families will normally meet a doctor and a nurse in the initial meeting. The team members will start by introducing themselves, telling families how long the session will last and checking that they do not have any commitments that mean they will have to leave early. They outline what will happen during the session and reassure families that there is no need to go over all the problems in detail. The clinicians emphasise that their most important task is to explain to the family how the unit works so that together they can decide if the service has anything useful to offer the family.

Engaging with the child

The staff member will usually try to open the conversation by talking to the child about his favourite activities and interests and finding out what he is good at. This approach serves to start the meeting on a positive note and to avoid the danger of getting into a problem-focused discussion too soon. It also signals to the child and his parents that the staff value children and their views very highly, so much so that they want to hear from them first rather than their parents. This is an unusual situation for a child, who would often experience adults talking about him rather than to him.

Of course some children are very anxious about talking to adults – especially unfamiliar doctors and nurses – and if they do not want to talk after a few general and positive openings, the team would reassure them that it is also okay not to talk, and let them play and listen to the adults.

If they are able to manage to answer a few questions about positive areas of their life, then the team would ask them about their family and then move on to finding out what they had been told about coming to the unit. It is often very revealing to hear if parents have been able to explain to the child why he is coming to the centre in a way that the child can understand and go along with. This also gives the team a chance to hear from the child how he views the difficulties.

Talking with parents

When the team start to talk to the adults in the family they will also try to start with the positives: 'What is going well with…X at the moment?', 'What is Y really good at and what does he enjoy doing?', 'Tell us about the last time you and Z had some especially nice time together.' Again this approach helps to establish a positive theme to the discussion and reinforces to the children that the Croft team know that there are good things about them as well as some difficulties. Some parents find this approach very hard, as, understandably, they are very keen to tell the team all of the problems they are experiencing. They might feel that the professionals will not appreciate how difficult their lives are, but the interviewer will reassure parents that the staff want to find out about those areas too, and explain that if the family decide to take up the opportunity to come to the unit, there will be plenty of opportunities to discuss the difficulties in detail. This initial approach draws on principles from solution-focused therapy (SFT) (de Shazer *et al.* 1986), with an emphasis on uncovering strengths and a belief that the patient or client already has the tools to change his life for the better.

Beliefs and expectations

A very important part of this first meeting is exploring how the family view the problems they are experiencing and assessing how closely their understanding agrees or disagrees with the referring team.

Towards the end of the interview the team will ask parents what they want to change in their lives and how that might fit with the programme the team offer.

When asked 'What do you want out of an intervention?' many parents will say, 'For X to be happy', 'For Y to do what he is told', 'For someone to tell me what is going on in Z's mind'. It is then useful to try to distil these rather general aspirations into more specific targets: so, for instance, the interviewer might ask if X was happier, what would they be doing differently and what would be different in the family. This honing process can help everyone start to think about the aims of an intervention. This is the beginning of making a therapeutic contract with the family, a process that continues throughout their stay and often goes through a number of renegotiations!

At this point the team will often start to describe the programme to the family and explain what is on offer and what is asked of families. The team will try to be as realistic as possible in regard to what can be achieved so that families are not under the impression that an inpatient stay will result in a miraculous change in their child or their family difficulties. Most of the children who come to the service have chronic difficulties and it would be unfair to suggest that these would be resolved completely in a matter of six to eight weeks. On the other hand, families need to hear that change is possible, and with commitment on all sides positive differences can be achieved which will lead to a substantial improvement in their child's (and their family's) quality of life.

The therapeutic contract

Once the team have established that a referral is appropriate it is always the parents' choice whether they accept an admission or not. The team will have looked at the information from the referring agencies to establish that an initial meeting is appropriate before it is offered, so the decision about whether to proceed or not ultimately falls to the family. Sometimes families are under considerable pressure to accept – this might come from a health team who are struggling to work with a family or to know what to do next, from the child's school if his behaviour in school is very challenging, or from a social care team if there are high levels of concern about the child's level of care.

However anxious or eager professionals are for an assessment to take place, the team will not coerce a family into an admission. It is a major undertaking to ask a family to stay in an institution for some weeks, away from their own home and community, and to do so against their will is likely to be unproductive and could even be very harmful.

Assessing parenting

Some families start their work with the service as reluctant participants. This is particularly the case when one of the admission aims is to assess parenting capacity. Parents in this situation are aware that if they do not take up the offer of an admission they may find themselves in statutory processes such as legal proceedings to determine if they are fit to retain their parental responsibility for their children. Even in this very difficult situation the team work hard to find targets for intervention that both they and the parents find meaningful and acceptable.

Prior to undertaking a parenting capacity assessment the team will meet the professionals already involved with a family to hear about the current concerns and relevant background information. Most importantly, a network meeting enables different professionals to share their own views and for disagreements to be aired. The output of such a meeting should be a shared agreement about the areas of concern, the aims of an assessment and clarity about how the assessment will influence the child protection plan.

There are many different approaches to assessing parenting. In the UK child protection teams usually work within the Framework for Assessment (DH 2000) and the unit uses this framework too. Figure 2.1 below shows the domain of assessment. The three main areas are shown on the sides of the triangle: the child's developmental needs, parenting capacity and family and environmental factors.

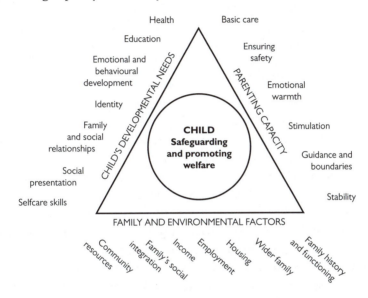

Figure 2.1 Framework for assessment

For a thorough assessment of all three sides of the triangle, a number of different professional perspectives are needed; for example, an educationalist would have valuable information on the child's developmental axis as would a paediatrician or child psychiatrist. A family therapist's viewpoint would be very valuable when considering the family factors influencing the child's world and close observation of parent–child interactions in a number of settings would be necessary to assess parenting capacity. For these reasons a child and family inpatient unit is well situated to undertake this very important and highly challenging work, and whilst most of these assessments are undertaken by community professionals, in the most complex and often contentious situations there is great value in a multi-disciplinary one-stop team who can encompass all three axes and consider the interplay between their strengths and deficits. In addition a mental health professional has specialist skills to assess the mental health of the parent and to consider how the parents' own emotional wellbeing is impacting on their care-giving.

Parents undergoing this assessment will be observed in everyday activities with their children as well as in more structured play or music sessions. The parenting care plan is based on a model suggested by Barker and Modes (2004). There is particular attention given to the children's behaviours that are most evident at times of separation, reunion and stress, as this can give clues to their attachment patterns (discussed further in Chapter 4).

Parenting capacity is not a dichotomous concept: good enough versus not good enough. Some children are temperamentally challenging or they may have particular disorders (such as attention deficit hyperactivity disorder (ADHD), autism or a learning disability) that make the parenting task much more challenging. In some families the parenting of one child can be quite adequate whereas another child's needs are not being met. So parenting capacity is assessed in relation to each child.

Understandably parents are very distressed by such an assessment due to its implicitly critical nature, but by maintaining a high level of respect for a family's view of the situation and acknowledging their reservations, often the team can work together with the family through the initial anxious and reluctant stage to establish a more trusting and productive working relationship.

What about families who say 'no'?

A small number of the families who are referred decide not to go ahead with an admission after they have come to an initial meeting. This may be because the practical logistics of attending for such a demanding admission are too difficult or because they do not feel the whole family approach would be useful. On some occasions just the threat of an admission can be helpful in moving a situation on. Community clinicians have described situations that have been very difficult and worrying and when they suggest an inpatient admission as the next step, then the child or family suddenly achieve an unexpected positive change!

Olivia is a ten-year-old girl; her family were very worried about her because her weight had dropped by three kilos in six weeks. She was severely restricting her diet and was resisting any pressure by her parents or outpatient team to reverse this. Her physical wellbeing was of concern; her blood pressure was low and her heartbeat slower than usual. She was complaining of feeling the cold and her concentration on her school work had deteriorated markedly. She refused to accept she had an eating problem and was refusing to be weighed or go to the clinic appointments.

The consultant psychiatrist in charge of her care was very worried and suggested that Olivia needed to have an inpatient admission to regain weight and re-establish normal eating patterns. Both Olivia and her parents were horrified at the suggestion, and concerned about how much school she would miss and how she would cope mixing with children with such a range of difficulties. Olivia begged for some time to show she did not need to go to hospital. The psychiatrist agreed to delay the referral for two weeks, insisting that she attend clinic and agree to be weighed.

Over the next two weeks Olivia's family became more insistent that she eat and she managed to increase her food input. She started to attend her clinic appointments and her weight started to creep up. She agreed to see a psychologist to discuss her difficulties with food and it was agreed that an admission could be put on hold.

Summary

This chapter has described the key features of the initial phase of engagement between the inpatient team and the family. Gathering and giving information, offering a warm welcome and a positive, respectful approach all contribute to getting the welcome right. This allows the team to establish a therapeutic contract with the family, forming the foundation of a working relationship as the family move into the challenging first few weeks of their admission. The contract will change, quite possibly a number of times over the weeks, but if the relationship between staff and family members is trusting and respectful, then these challenges can be met head on and used to promote the positive change everyone is working towards.

The next two chapters consider the very important areas of containment and nurturing, which form the foundation for therapeutic assessment and intervention.

Chapter 3

Structure and Containment

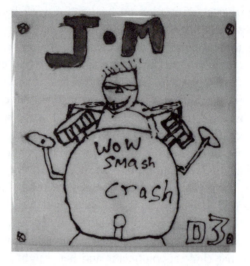

Playing the drums was a fantastic outlet for J.M.

The therapeutic frame

Children who require inpatient admission present with complex and severe difficulties that cannot adequately be assessed and treated in community settings alone. Often the reason that community intervention is not sufficient is that the family have reached a crisis point where the structure of everyday life has broken down. This could be because the child is not attending school, is refusing to eat or is being violent to family members. It could be that parents are in conflict about how to manage their child, or parents could be separating or physically unwell. Whatever the reason, the consequence is that the usual routines of work, school, mealtimes and bedtimes are lost and life has become chaotic and directionless. In this situation family activity becomes focused on the here and now and energies are directed towards reducing and avoiding distress and anxiety. It becomes difficult to formulate plans and to think beyond the problems of the moment.

An inpatient admission provides an environment that can both help to rebuild that structure and assess and treat the underlying cause of the breakdown. The assessment and treatments provided in inpatient units are broadly similar to those that are offered in outpatient clinics and the same clinicians frequently work in both settings. The difference between community and inpatient setting is the context or therapeutic frame in which the work takes place.

The therapeutic frame refers to the physical environment and the daily life of the service: the hours of business, the composition of the staff team, the therapeutic programme, the rules and boundaries and how these are applied, how everyday tasks are attended to, the staff support and supervision structures, the interaction with external agencies, clinical governance arrangements and safeguarding and legislation.

The frame not only provides a context for assessment and treatment to take place but can also be therapeutic in its own right. It is an intervention that can treat structural problems in family life. Maintaining the frame is usually a core task of the nursing team as they manage the day-to-day running of the unit and provide the majority of face-to-face contact with children and parents. This element of care is often invisible and unacknowledged, and this is especially true when it is working well! But like the glue that holds a structure together, if it fails the effects are immediate and can create chaos and anxiety. Some of the important principles of the creation and maintenance of the therapeutic frame are illustrated by events during Nick and Stacey's first week of admission.

> When Nick and his mother Stacey were referred to the Croft it seemed that all aspects of their lives were dysfunctional; there appeared to be no domain that was ordinary or free from stress. Nick did not attend school and Stacey had had to give up work and had no social life. The usual hierarchies and boundaries of family life were disrupted, Nick was in charge at home, his mother had no authority over him and she was scared of his violence and aggression. Stacey had abandoned normal expectations of behaviour in favour of accommodating to Nick's agenda in order to

avoid arousing heightened states of emotion leading to fearful and out of control situations.

Nick, aged 11, was socialising with an older delinquent peer group of 15- to 17-year-olds and had started to get into trouble with the police. He had a reversed sleep pattern and insisted on sleeping in his mother's bed. Moreover Nick was very unhappy, suffered panic attacks and was deliberately harming himself. Like many parents seen in child and adolescent mental health (CAMH) services Stacey described a situation in which her family had drifted so far away from accepted norms that she did not know how to get back into a situation of ordinary family life.

The community psychiatrist feared that Nick would become involved in the criminal justice system, which he believed would be detrimental and inappropriate. Different approaches had been tried by agencies in the community, but Nick's risky behaviour continued to escalate despite concerted efforts. As an emergency measure he had been prescribed medication to reduce his level of arousal and anxiety, and whilst Stacey reported that this had taken the edge off his anger, it was of concern that he was taking medication at such a young age and this could only be used as a short-term measure.

A period at a boarding school had failed as Nick's distress was so extreme because he could not tolerate being separated from his mother and constantly absconded to get back to her. At the Croft it was hoped that Nick and his mother could receive treatment together and that separation from his mother could be undertaken in a gradual way once Nick had started to develop trusting relationships with staff.

The Croft team knew that admitting Nick would be difficult and would provoke high levels of anxiety for both him and his mother. Staff needed to be prepared to manage high risk behaviours including violence and aggression, self-harm and absconding. It would undoubtedly involve the team in imposing boundaries on Nick's current levels of unfettered behaviour, which Stacey would need to sanction.

There had been some discussion as to whether Nick should be treated in an adolescent service as his behaviours were more typical of a 15- or 16-year-old; he was sexually active, smoking, drinking, self-harming and carrying weapons. However, following the principle of trying to reinstitute normal expectations and routines, the team felt that in the first instance Nick should be given the opportunity to conform to the usual norms of his chronological age. It was thought that if he was treated as though he were an older teenager, it would be harder to establish whether or not he was able to allow himself to behave as a child.

The structure

Most inpatient units draw upon theoretical principles that have been developed in therapeutic communities. These communities developed after the Second World War, partly in response to the recognition that the large psychiatric asylums built in Victorian times were inappropriate for soldiers returning from the war with post-traumatic stress disorders such as shell shock. Cassel Hospital in London is one of the original therapeutic communities, and in addition to a strong psychodynamic basis to group therapy, their programme emphasises the importance of psychosocial nursing and a living–learning therapeutic environment. The loss of daily structure and family functioning continues to be an important focus for treatment. Roger Kennedy from Cassel Hospital writes that 'the hospital can provide a holding and facilitating environment in which families can attempt to restore their functioning and so return to ordinary life' (Kennedy, Heymans and Tischler 1987). Thus the family can utilise the hospital's structure as a kind of scaffolding as they rebuild their own.

The central scaffolding at the Croft is the unit programme and the rules and boundaries that the staff uphold. At the Croft there are three parallel and interconnected programmes: for children, parents (see Appendices 4 and 5) and staff. These programmes provide a containing structure that aims to meet the needs of each group in a coherent and planned way.

Nick's first day

On his first night at the Croft Nick reluctantly went to his bedroom at 10 p.m. when he realised that the staff were going to stand firm about the television being switched off. He was awake until about 1 a.m. playing games on his mother's phone. Although he was given his own room he dragged his mattress into Stacey's room, and she reported that Nick usually insists on sleeping with her when he eventually retires at 3 a.m. and her partner then has to spend the rest of the night in Nick's bed. Stacey was very tense and said that she was surprised he didn't kick off and thought he was getting the measure of the staff before revealing his true colours.

In the morning Nick remained in bed whilst the other families busied themselves getting ready for the day. June, a member of the nursing team, suggested that Stacey wake Nick so that he could be ready for the programme at 9 a.m. Stacey was reluctant to do this as she was anxious that it would provoke him. June suggested that she have a go and Stacey agreed but appeared anxious. June opened Nick's door and suggested that he come and have some breakfast and then join the other children for morning meeting. Nick swore at her and buried his head in his pillow. When the other children had left the residential area Nick appeared, looking grumpy and wrapped in his duvet. He walked towards the television but was prevented from turning it on by Andrew (nurse) who stated that the television was not allowed on during programme time. Nick swore and returned to his room, kicking objects and pulling down a curtain rail on his way. Stacey burst into tears and apologised to parents and staff and said she was mortified by his behaviour. She was terrified he would kick off and hurt someone. She also expressed a concern that the staff might be punitive and was afraid that he would be put in the soft room. The firm but gentle prompts and boundaries given by June and Andrew seemed to have been experienced by Stacey as highly provocative and dangerous. We later learnt from family therapy that Stacey and Nick had both experienced considerable violence from Nick's biological father during his infancy. Stacey had also experienced abuse in her own infancy.

Children's timetable

For the children there is a daily timetable of activities that runs from 9 a.m. to 3.30 p.m. that deliberately aims to mirror an ordinary school day. The children attend the unit school in the morning and therapeutic groups in the afternoons. The content of the sessions is described further in later chapters.

Many of the children who come to the Croft have had serious difficulties in school settings and often arrive at the unit having either not attended school at all for months or having attended for just a few hours a week. Consequently starting a daily programme with a group of peers can be highly challenging. The children often arrive with an expectation that their difficult behaviour with teachers will lead to them returning to the care of their parents and to the disappearance of whatever demand has triggered their behaviour. At the Croft this does not happen – when children display challenging behaviour this is dealt with and then the children are expected to return to the daily programme and to complete the day. This reinforces the message that adults can manage these difficulties, that negative emotions or behaviours can be resolved and that ordinary routines can carry on.

The rules, rewards and sanctions

During the daily programme children are with their peers and are supervised by the staff team. The children are introduced to the rules of the unit as soon as they arrive and there are frequent reminders of these at the beginning of almost every activity (see Appendix 1). It is made clear to the children that the rules are there to keep everyone safe and to allow everyone to enjoy their time.

There are timely behavioural rewards and sanctions built into the programme to encourage children to keep on track. For instance, after a session of education or group therapy there is always a break during which the children have a drink and free playtime. If any child has transgressed the rules during the group session she will have to wait quietly in the therapy room for a few minutes at the end of the session before she can join her peers in the playground. This is called 'making up minutes'. Children can earn back these minutes during the group with good behaviour.

The team put huge amounts of effort into creating opportunities for success for the children as most arrive at the unit with extremely low self-esteem and an expectation of failure and rejection. The staff make liberal use of praise – there are big smiles and cries of 'well done' if a child manages even a small achievement. For some children that might mean managing to line up with other children without hitting someone, or telling an adult that they are upset. All children are given a specific task for the week (see Appendix 2). The team aim to foster an environment in which adults make it easy for children to find ways out of difficulties, to resolve conflicts and to move on to something positive. An important part of the work is to pass on this experience and approach to parents who also arrive at the unit, like their children, with expectations of failure and criticism of their efforts.

Containing aggression

Aggression is a very common feature of children with complex emotional and behavioural difficulties. For some children this forms part of a pattern of a conduct disorder when it is accompanied by a number of other antisocial behaviours such as stealing, absconding or cruelty to animals. For other children their aggression may be a response to anxiety and a way of controlling their environment. If this aggression is severe and high frequency it can paralyse the adults around the child and prevent change. Reversing this dynamic is essential to re-establish adult authority, thus reassuring the children that adults can be in charge and can manage their distress.

A key part of the training for staff working closely with children with severe mental health difficulties is the management of aggression. There are a number of different training programmes used in health, education and social care provisions in the UK, and they all share common themes: early identification of trigger situations, de-escalation techniques, safe physical containment and post-incident debriefing. At the Croft a programme developed in the USA at the Crisis Prevention Institute (CPI) is used (CPI Nonviolent Crisis Intervention programme, see www.crisisprevention.co.uk).

In situations when a child is becoming angry, staff will use humour or distraction to try to divert the child and to reduce her negative arousal; they will also remind her of activities she will be able to do if she is calm. If this is not successful and the child's aggression becomes a risk to herself or others, then the staff will move the child to a quiet area (or move the other children away to another area). A quiet non-stimulating room where the child cannot find ways to hurt herself or others can be very helpful in calming down. The unit has a soft room which has cushion padding on the walls and flooring and soft cushions that the child can use to throw around or build a den. The staff can see the child at all times and can monitor her level of emotional arousal; as she calms down, the staff will re-engage verbally with the child, offering her a drink. Once she is calm the child will rejoin the other children or her parents. During her time in the soft room the child's parents will be informed and will be invited to join the staff in monitoring the child and thinking of ways to help the child calm down. This gives an opportunity for staff to model a calm authoritative response to the child's aggression. An example of a care plan for managing difficult behaviour is given in Appendix 3.

The challenge of separation

Many children using the service are very anxious about being apart from their parent or primary carer, and this anxiety usually has complex roots. But it is an important issue that often needs to be tackled early on in an admission if children are to be able to access the therapeutic opportunities available for them. As discussed in Chapter 2, a focus on positive engagement with the child is key, establishing a trusting relationship and approaching this separation in a sensitive and gradual way. It has been observed that this is a more successful approach for children for whom this is a chronic problem than trying to separate parent and child in a sudden and dramatic way. Too rapid a separation might lead to a child merely transferring her anxious adhesive attachment to a member of staff rather than developing her tolerance of being away from her primary attachment figure in a more positive and sustainable way.

In an unpublished piece of research (Kenny 2001) it was observed that adolescents in this situation who were admitted to an adolescent inpatient unit often showed an escalating pattern of risky behaviour that resulted in them requiring intensive nursing.

> For reasons that were initially uncertain Nick became highly anxious when he was not with Stacey and feared that she was unsafe. He spent the first couple of days on the unit with his mother getting to know staff and the other residents. Although initially he was adamant that he would not leave Stacey, he gradually joined in with staff and other children in games in the evenings. On day three staff felt that he would really like to spend more time with the other children as he was getting bored just sitting with his mum watching television all day. Both his key worker and Stacey encouraged him to give the programme a try and he agreed to join the other children on the daily programme on the proviso that his mum stayed on the unit and that he could check in with her at regular intervals.

Initially Nick went out of activities every 15 minutes to see Stacey briefly – over the first couple of weeks the frequency of this was gradually decreased to every 30 minutes and then every hour. By the end of week three Nick was forgetting to ask staff if he could go and see his mum and he agreed that he could manage the whole day programme without seeing her.

Stacey told staff that previously if she ever tried to go out or leave Nick with someone else he would make such a fuss that she had tended to sneak away when he was distracted. Unfortunately over time this had caused him to be even more anxious and vigilant about her whereabouts and not to trust what she said about what she was doing.

A key worker organised for Stacey to have planned time away from Nick whilst he was on the unit. She was supported in telling Nick when she was leaving the unit and for how long. At first each time she left he became very upset and angry but staff helped him to cope with these feelings. They found activities for him to do when his mum was out and praised him for coping so well. Over the weeks Nick became much more able to cope when Stacey left the unit and he even asked to have a couple of nights on the unit on his own during the last week. Whilst playing pool with one of his key workers one evening he said how good it felt not to have to worry about his mum so much.

Structure for parents

A predictable and containing structure is also important for parents. The parent groups are based on the Mellow Parenting programme (Puckering 2004) which advises that intervention needs to target three domains to provide the best outcomes. These are: parenting skills which are addressed in the behaviour management group, the quality of the relationship between parent and child which is addressed in the Mellow Parenting group and the parent's own needs as an individual adult which are addressed in the parents' support group. As well as the groups, each family is offered family therapy once a week, and they will have individual sessions with members of the team as appropriate to the care plan. Additional groups target the parent's own wellbeing, such as the parents' support group and the parents' yoga group.

Parents often feel daunted by what seems like a lot of spare time in their timetable, and it is striking how many parents express a need to keep busy to keep unpleasant thoughts and feelings at bay. It is not unusual for parents to spend time cleaning the unit kitchen or cooking in the first couple of weeks. Staff offer ideas of how parents can occupy their time but also take the opportunity to think with parents about how their lives have become dominated by caring for their children and how they can regain their own sense of themselves.

The integrated model of care

Inpatient treatment can be conceptualised as being either bipolar or integrated. In the bipolar model there is a strict divide between a therapeutic space, where therapies take place, and a social space, in which patients are nursed and gather together for social activities. In the integrated model, all levels of interaction are seen as therapeutic and considered as a whole (Ward *et al.* 2003).

An integrated service offers more than just an outpatient treatment with beds and more than just care and containment. This type of group care involves processes in which the integrated model is used and where there is a close interdependence of team members. There is also a co-ordinated and therapeutic use of the routines of daily living and opportunity-led work that makes therapeutic use of the informal everyday life of the unit (Ward *et al.* 2003).

This approach is most in evidence during the residential programme, the time between the ending of the day programme at 3.15 p.m. and its restart the following day at 9 a.m. The rules and boundaries regarding behaviour, bedtimes and mealtimes, whilst designed to mirror ordinary expectations, are often vastly different from how families coming to the Croft actually function. During this time the children are returned to the supervision of their parents supported by the nursing team. Parents have the opportunity to try out different strategies for managing their child's problems with the close support of nursing staff. The structure is not rigid but is a flexible and sensitive instrument that can be adapted to meet the needs of each child and family.

Children with complex emotional needs often struggle to use the formal settings in which assessment and treatment usually occur, so working in an integrated way enables the work to happen as and when the opportunity arrives. The functioning of daily life is often the arena for assessments to take place rather than just the background support for formal work. For instance, how a family manage mealtimes or how a child copes with a bedtime routine often provides a great insight into family functioning, and this can complement information gleaned in family therapy sessions or other more formal therapy settings.

Whilst the nursing team will work to establish a clear structure and place boundaries on children's behaviour, other members of the multi-disciplinary team will be closely involved in observing and consulting roles.

If a child's behaviour is posing a high risk then the nursing team may have to institute a restriction of that child's liberty, but the medical team has the responsibility to review this and to work jointly with the nursing team to ensure that such restrictions are used appropriately and for the shortest possible time. The unit has a well-documented restriction of liberty policy that has evolved over many years.

> Nick was not able to tolerate being in a therapy room on his own, for formal assessments and therapies, so until the third week of his admission assessment relied on detailed observations of his functioning on the group programme and in the residential setting.
>
> Initially staff needed to pick their battles, and in the initial stages they only addressed the most risky behaviours whilst trying to build a relationship with the family and engage Nick in the programme. So in week one the issues of Nick smoking with his mother, sleeping in her bed, and having chocolate bars and fizzy drinks for breakfast were not addressed. The team aim to establish a respectful relationship and try to learn more about his anxiety when separated from his mother and work gently to get him into the unit programme. The community rules of the unit need to be maintained, for example times when television is allowed on, and the team also have to intervene in any behaviour that may cause a risk to himself or others. Staff let him know what is expected of him and encourage him to join the programme. The team capitalise on his interest in motorbikes and try to create positive opportunities for him. Despite this Stacey remained very concerned that Nick would be enraged by the mild restrictions imposed on him and 'kick off'. An advantage that the staff team have over parents is the

ability to follow through behavioural consequences and remain in charge, through the co-ordinated use of the team and the facilities available in the building. For some children, including Nick, this means that for the first time in a long while they will not be able to control the people around them through the use of violence and aggression.

It is a firm belief that at the Croft, admissions have the best chance of a successful outcome if they are carefully prepared. In Nick's case a nurse met with his mother at a pre-admission visit to get a detailed picture of his behavioural difficulties, potential triggers and useful ways of managing the difficulties. His mother, Stacey, reported that the only way she could manage was to let Nick be in control and have his own way. She admitted soothing him by giving him cigarettes and letting him share her bed. She reported that he responds to behavioural consequences with bravado and was insolent to police officers when arrested. There was some evidence in old school reports, however, that he did respond to rewards and praise. Stacey was able to say that he could be very kind and thoughtful, particularly to younger children. She said that he had a passion for motorbikes and loved tinkering with engines. She was visibly anxious at the thought that the Croft team might try to impose boundaries on Nick and expressed the fear that something catastrophic would happen. She was afraid that Nick would be angry with her if she allowed staff to be in charge and he would vent this anger when they were at home at the weekend.

In the weekly group supervision discussion meeting prior to Nick's arrival the multi-disciplinary team discussed how the team should best manage the risks that Nick posed and an initial care plan was made. The team decided to pay equal attention to supporting Stacey and to developing a way of working that would help to move Nick into the therapeutic structure but would not cause such intolerable levels of distress that Stacey would decide to leave.

It was clear that Nick and Stacey's difficulties were complex and needed a multi-modal and intensive intervention to effect any significant change. The most pressing problem was the lack of structure and boundaries to their lives, leading to dangerously out of control situations.

Multi-modal treatment model

Inpatient treatment is multi-modal and allows difficulties to be addressed at different levels simultaneously. Theories about the nature and meaning of mental health and behavioural difficulties range from the physiological to societal, and can be described in a number of domains, which include:

- *The physical domain* refers to factors that relate to the physical constitution of the child; her genetic make-up, biochemistry, the presence or absence of physical conditions, for example, epilepsy, learning disability, mental illness and also the individual's sensory profile; and what soothes or stimulates her level of emotional arousal. History taking would establish any history of head injury, exposure to toxins in utero, and so on. Intervention at this level could include prescription of medication, assessing learning level, blood tests, electroencephalograms or brain scans.

  > Nick had been prescribed stimulant medication by the community psychiatrist in the hope that it would reduce his level of over-arousal. There were mixed views about whether this had been helpful and Nick complained that the medication made him feel 'weird'. During Nick's second week at the unit the team decided to reduce his medication gradually to re-evaluate the impact it was having on his symptoms. The unit doctor discussed this with Stacey – she was initially reluctant to consider a trial off medication but was reassured that the reduction would be done gradually. Blood tests were also taken to establish if he had been taking any illicit substances or had any other biochemical abnormalities. As the medication was reduced the team used structured observation sheets to record his levels of over-activity, distractability and impulsivity.

- *The intra-psychic domain* refers to the individual's internal world, the meanings and attributions that the individual attaches to the world around her and how she responds to them. The team is attending to this domain when the child or parent's beliefs about themselves and others, their self-esteem, their emotional state and the meaning of their responses and behaviour are considered. Clinicians intervene by trying to achieve change through an understanding of the individual's internal world, for example, by identifying rewards that will motivate a child and being sensitive to factors that would soothe rather than further distress an individual child, for example, by understanding their preference for proximity or distance when angry or aroused. Staff can intervene in individual work with the child or parent through counselling or through play.

> Nick would not take part in formal individual sessions but during informal play he showed very aggressive themes in his fantasy life. His internal landscape was akin to a war-torn city; he operated as though life was a constant fight for survival in which there was danger at every turn. Any unexpected noise would make him jump out of his skin. He was constantly plagued with the idea that his mother was unsafe; he found it hard to separate from her and needed to control her when he was with her.

- *The interpersonal domain* refers to the impact of relationships on a child's functioning. Staff consider the characteristics and quality of important relationships including areas of strength as well as areas of difficulty. In this domain the attachment patterns of the child and the parents are important considerations. Attachment theory is discussed in more detail in the next chapter. Staff intervene at this level formally in family therapy sessions and in dyadic music or play therapy sessions.

> As the admission progressed Stacey became more relaxed and open. She revealed that she had been abused as a child and had a series of abusive partners, including Nick's father, as an adult. She had suffered with depression throughout her life, had made several suicide attempts and on one occasion Nick had had to call for help when she had overdosed. During Nick's first couple of years of life she was regularly physically abused by his father. She felt that she was depressed and at home she often drank alcohol or used cannabis to cope with her low mood.

At this level the team works with parents to help them develop a more effective approach to their child's difficulties and to encourage a more secure and trusting relationship. The staff have to examine their own part in the work by thinking about the transference and counter-transference processes – the emotions and relationship patterns recreated in the children, parents and staff which have their origin in earlier experiences in their lives.

> There was a tight and intense bond between Nick and his mother, driven by his belief that she was unsafe and that something might happen to her if he was not around. Nick was suspicious of actions taken by the team that created distance between himself and his mother. He often seemed older than his peers and had a rather adult way of relating that was incongruent with his actual age. He was particularly anxious about male members of staff especially if he saw them talking to his mother. He would sometimes accuse them of trying to chat her up. He would be hostile and rejecting of male staff members. This was upsetting to the staff members involved but they used their supervision sessions to think about Nick's experiences of rejection by his own father and the fear he must have experienced watching his mother's physical abuse. This helped them to realise why Nick was so negative towards them. Their patience and acceptance of Nick's negative feelings helped Nick to gradually build relationships with the male members of staff. In fact Nick became especially attached to one male member of staff, and towards the end of his stay he would always ask if he was on duty and seek him out to play pool or build LEGO® models.

The physical environment

In addition to considering children's physical functioning, their psychological functioning and their interpersonal functioning, it is also important to consider their relationship to their wider environment. When they are living at home this would include the quality of their neighbourhood, their school and the places they visit for leisure activities. Aspects of this wider environment can facilitate mental wellbeing or impair it. For instance, children with autism spectrum conditions often have problems processing and filtering sensory stimuli in their environment – they may become overwhelmed by excessive noise or even too many pieces of artwork on a wall. Thus, when planning learning environments for these children, consideration has to be given to sensory overload.

In a setting for children with complex needs, a balance has to be struck between a homely, normative environment and a setting where children can be easily supervised and risky behaviour managed safely. For some families being inside the unit can often create feelings of emotional and physical safety that they have not experienced for a long time.

The building itself has obvious safety features: there is a safe, low stimulus garden as well as a garden with playground equipment. There is a soft room that is used for time out and physical containment of risky behaviour, but it is also used for fun and rough play. There are high handles to the doors to slow down children who might be trying to run out of the building. All sharp objects such as knives are kept locked away and staff are constantly monitoring the environment for any item that might be dangerous. Whilst these are procedures that have to happen in an institutional setting to ensure safety, they can stimulate parents to think about safety in their own homes and how they might adjust their environments to keep their children and themselves safe. In addition to reducing hazards, the unit also places a high value on positive activities such as craft, music, outdoor play or toys that stimulate imaginative play since keeping children active and engaged improves their self-esteem and mood and reduces the risk of maladaptive behaviours.

There is something about the actual building that has meaning for the child and family and it is often referred to. This could be because the place is associated with mainly positive experiences, or because it is spacious, bright, and child and family friendly. Children often want to visit the building after discharge and want to wander around, looking in the various rooms and reliving their experiences.

The evening plan

The team encourage parents to plan their evenings with their children to encourage structure and positive activity. This also creates an opportunity for discussion and negotiation between the child and parent. If parents have lost their sense of authority over their child because of the child's severe problems (or possibly because of their own depression or anxiety) then sitting down together to decide when to have tea and when to play a board game may be the start of re-negotiating the parent–child relationship.

> At home Nick was used to 'doing his own thing'. He would order Stacey to make his tea whenever he felt hungry, he would leave the house as he chose and return likewise. He was in charge of the remote control of the television and Stacey had to ask him if she could watch her favourite soap operas.
>
> On Nick's first evening on the unit he completely refused to sit with Stacey and his key worker to make a plan. Despite this the key worker encouraged Stacey to put together a plan that they stuck up on the wall alongside the plans for the other children. Stacey told Nick when tea would be. Nick swore at her and told her he would eat when he wanted. The key worker reiterated the rule that the children were not allowed to help themselves to food and encouraged Stacey to make tea at the time she had said. Stacey felt that it would be useless and that she was likely to get a plate of food thrown at her. However, the key worker helped Stacey to prepare the meal and they called Nick to the dining room. Initially he refused and started kicking chairs around the room – the staff reminded him that if he continued he would have to go to his room to calm down. Nick then started throwing toys around the room, narrowly missing staff and another parent. Staff took Nick to his room for time out; meanwhile Nick's key worker talked to Stacey, reassuring her that Nick was okay and that he would calm down. Half an hour later Nick was calm in his room – he told staff he was hungry and they took him to eat with his mum in the dining room. Later Stacey told her key worker it was the first time she and Nick had sat at a table to eat together since he was six.

Community living

Another important factor in a communal environment is the amount of social contact within the community. Many families with children with special needs experience social isolation and exclusion. They cannot take their children to the supermarket or the local swimming pool because of their challenging behaviour. Often they lose friends who stop coming to visit because they do not want to be involved in a family that is struggling with so many problems. Parents become more and more housebound and in some situations may even develop their own anxiety about going out.

A communal setting where a number of families are sharing space can be very stressful and challenging for families but it can force parents and children back into social interaction, thus re-establishing their confidence and, it is hoped, enjoyment in this area. This social community setting can also be utilised to assist children to re-engage with ordinary daily activities such as eating with the family or having a set bedtime. Children generally want to interact with their peers and if their peers are going to a music group or into school, the social pressure for a reluctant child to accompany them may well help that child to overcome her anxiety.

In a community situation families have the opportunity to learn vicariously by seeing what other families are doing and this in turn can make them reflect on their own parenting in a different way. Joint family work is discussed in more detail in Chapter 5.

> Stacey saw other children, younger than Nick, managing to separate from their parents and enjoying being in group activities. This helped her have confidence that Nick could also achieve this. Other parents encouraged her to work with the staff when they suggested gradually increasing Nick's time away from her, and although she felt very anxious about doing this, the support of her new-found friends tipped the balance. When Nick realised that it was not just the unit staff encouraging him to join the programme but that his mother also agreed that it was a good idea, his resistance began to weaken. Through talking with staff and other parents, and seeing other children on the programme, Stacey also came to accept that placing boundaries on Nick's behaviour was not going to permanently damage her relationship with him or his mental state.

Research shows that the earlier a child is exposed to extreme fear and not protected, the more likely it is that the brain function becomes set to experience even mildly frightening events as highly dangerous. Tiny triggers can then set off major fear responses or rage as a biological form of self-protection (Ward *et al.* 2003).

As described above, ways of avoiding these triggers are inherent in some of the routines of the Croft. For example, the children meet at the beginning of every day to hear about the day's structure. If they then have an individual meeting with a therapist later in the day, it will not come as a shock or a surprise. This attempt to increase predictability in otherwise chaotic lives is important. Similarly, at the end of each day the children review their day. This also helps to put some structure into their lives as well as encouraging some degree of reflection. In addition parents are encouraged to construct some sort of plan of activities with their children after the school day. The Croft also has rules, for example, after 8.30 p.m. children are encouraged to spend quiet time in their rooms.

> Over the course of the admission, working on these issues, Nick calmed down and became more compliant as he built a therapeutic relationship with staff. He felt increasingly contained and safe with them and began to trust they would look after his mum. Stacey also became emotionally stronger and more assertive. She was encouraged to give Nick space, and to be selective in her battles with him.
>
> Nick was also gradually introduced into school by encouraging his mother to separate from him during the day in graded ways. At each transition he wanted to return to her. Staff helped Stacey to calibrate her distance from him in the first few days. At first she wanted to be too close by, looking through a window into school so that Nick could see her. Then in contrast, the next day, she left the unit without letting Nick know. There were planned reunions during the day; so, for instance, Nick could spend a couple of minutes with Stacey in the midmorning break. Nick started to have more confidence that she would not disappear without telling him and he worried less.

Containing the containers: staff structures

Outside the programmes for children and parents the staff team have a number of structured meetings throughout the week. The aim of these meetings is to maintain the team's ability to work together effectively. Some meetings are mainly to exchange information and to formulate plans for the children and families, such as handover meetings and the weekly ward round.

In addition, there are two meetings each week in which there is space for the staff team to think and reflect on their practice. In group supervision there is an opportunity to discuss clinical issues in depth and to think about some of the complex dynamics that may be around. Often the space is used to think about a family who are due to arrive on the unit, to familiarise the team with the information that has been gathered and to create some ideas about how they might be approached. The space is also used to think about issues that staff are struggling to manage or understand. The staff support group at the end of the week is facilitated by an external group therapist. It is a time for the team to consider their own emotional response to the work they are doing and the impact it has on their relationships with the children, parents and each other. Both these groups are described in more detail in the next chapter, which deals with nurturing structures.

Working in a highly emotive environment there is an ever-present danger that the staff team will find themselves caught up in unhelpful behaviour that mirrors that of the families they work with, and that they lose their own structures and professional boundaries in the face of fierce primitive anxieties. In order to avoid this and to be able to work effectively, there are two spaces a week for the team to think together as a team as well as each member of staff having individual supervision.

Sometimes staff members will feel too busy to manage disturbance and at the same time keep the therapeutic programme in place. Opportunities to think and reflect are lost with the dual effect of staff being blindly organised by anxiety and being unable to think about what is happening to them. Organisational defences can emerge that, on the one hand, protect the team from experiencing uncomfortable emotions, but on the other, disrupt the team's ability to think sensitively about the work and to operate therapeutically. For example, staff may become focused on tasks that need to be completed rather than remaining alert to the emotional aspects of the work (Menzies Lyth 1988). Without these structures it is easy for staff to take the path of least resistance, to avoid anything that might increase anxiety even though that may not be therapeutic for the patient.

In an inpatient unit there are frequent staff meetings throughout the week. These include handovers at the start of each shift, a weekly patient review meeting, a referrals meeting and a staff reflection group. In other intensive services regular meetings and supervision will also be built into the programme to support staff in managing the complex dynamics that the work involves. In between these formal meeting the staff office serves as a vital space for staff to vent their feelings and to receive help and support from colleagues. In a well-functioning team expression of frustration or anger in a professional space should be encouraged, but alongside this there needs to be a culture of colleagues validating that experience and also helping staff members to process their emotions and to see where these feelings may be coming from, either as projections from very distressed children or parents or from their own experiences of conflict or distress. In either case, acknowledgement and acceptance of these feelings are vital to keep staff members emotionally balanced with the resources to continue to work productively with families.

> Nick's high level of anxiety was contagious, and during his first few days there were many discussions in the staff room about how much the team should be expecting of him and how much to encourage separation between Nick and his mother. Some staff were very sensitive to Nick's distress and were drawn to a very slow 'Nick-led' pace, whilst other staff members were impatient to see change and worried that allowing Nick to dictate the pace of separation might reinforce his sense of control over adults. There was a sense that staff were experiencing the contagion of Nick and Stacey's anxiety and were at risk of acting into it rather than containing it. The team might collude with Nick's controlling behaviours and let him set the agenda, and might adopt Stacey's stance of appeasing him to prevent conflict, thereby creating a situation of no change. Alternatively, if staff were too challenging, then Stacey and Nick might be so distressed that they would not be able to continue the work and abandon the admission. The charge nurse played a key role in listening to the concerns of various team members and respecting them – she called together a mini-team of the key workers, the unit doctor and psychologist, to discuss the dilemma and agree a plan. This was discussed with the wider team at handovers and during the weekly review. At the staff support meeting at the end of the week both sides of the argument were aired and it led on to a discussion about the hierarchy within the unit about who should have a voice and who should have a final say in decisions about a child's care plan.

This delicate way of working reflects concepts described by Bateson as the 'difference that makes the difference', encouraging families or systems to find the optimal level of change, when too small a difference evokes no change, and too great a difference stresses the relationship to breaking point (Bateson 1972).

In addition to internal structures to support staff there are external processes that are vital to ensure that the care delivered is effective and appropriate. The wider organisation undertakes audit and benchmarking activities so that the unit can consider their treatment alongside other similar mental health units. There are statutory regulatory bodies that visit and inspect the unit. The unit is also part of a national network of children's mental health units, so once again approaches to children can be compared and reviewed to ensure that any one unit does not become too idiosyncratic or out of step with mainstream care. These statutory regulatory bodies are referred to again in Chapter 11. In addition, the unit works with a national advocacy service to ensure that there is a neutral person who meets children to gain their perspective of their experience. This again helps the team to reflect on the work that they do and challenges them to change.

Summary

This chapter has described the broad therapeutic framework at the Croft and how this provides structure and containment for the children and families who are admitted. This is a particularly important foundation to the whole assessment and treatment process given the level of chaos that many families present with. The ideas presented around one specific case example of a child admitted to an inpatient unit would also apply to the care of children and families in other settings. Attending to structure and containing distress has to be tackled at the start of an intervention, otherwise attempts at specific therapies will never get off the ground. Providing support to people working with children and families in great distress has also been described, and again this is a vital element of maintaining an effective, healthy team. Without these structures teams will be plagued by low staff retention, high levels of sickness and low team cohesion and morale. And lastly, there is an important, often unacknowledged role for external monitoring of services. This may be seen as intrusive by teams but without it services are at risk of losing touch with the broader context of their work and becoming over-consumed by their own internal issues.

Running alongside structure and containment is the process of establishing positive relationships with children and families, and the next chapter goes on to explore how these relationships are nurtured.

Chapter 4

A Nurturing Environment

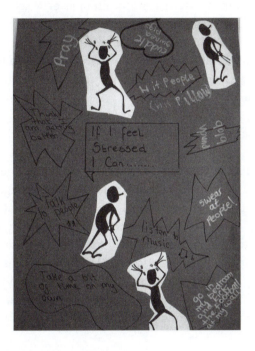

A child who discovered she could communicate her feelings

Introduction

In the parenting research literature discipline and nurturing are two of the most heavily researched constructs, but the ways of using them vary in both method and content (Locke and Prinz 2002). The previous chapter explored the issues of discipline whilst this chapter focuses on nurturing.

Nurturing is a multi-faceted concept, and frequently seen as a necessary, but not sufficient, aspect of parenting that contributes to the formation of secure attachments in children. In the context of the complex families who use child and adult mental health (CAMH) services, lack of nurturing is often a key issue, both in terms of the parenting that children are receiving and the care that parents experienced as children. Within inpatient or intensive mental health services, nurturing and containment combine to provide a safe and emotionally responsive therapeutic setting.

Nurturing can be viewed as an attitude, or a set of observable behaviours, that encompasses a broad range of feelings which can be innate, learned or enhanced with practice. The parental nurturing domain surrounds and scaffolds the child and needs to be supported and protected (Zeenah 2000) for the development of the child's emotional and social wellbeing.

Nurturing includes providing for basic needs and giving an appropriate level of protection from harm, such as neglect, abandonment, physical abuse or sexual abuse. A nurturing attitude would not deny, dominate or bully, but rather acknowledge and validate the individual. The aim would be to encourage self-esteem rather than belittle, to give consistency rather than unpredictability, to encourage social adaptation rather than dependency or deviancy, and to provide appropriate levels of stimulation for emotional and intellectual growth for the individual's level of development.

Obviously, therefore, a deficit of nurturing will lead to significant harm and is a fundamental aspect of the child protection categories of neglect and emotional abuse used in the UK (DH 2000).

Attachment theory

Attachment theory is one of the most important and influential theories in child mental health (British Psychological Society 2007), and is fundamental to the concept of nurturing. Bowlby first described attachment theory in the early 1950s, based on his work with delinquent youths and children who had experienced separation from their parents during hospital treatment. He stated that 'the infant and young child should experience a warm, intimate, and continuous relationship with his mother (or permanent mother substitute) in which both find satisfaction and enjoyment' (Bowlby 1951, p.13). Mary Ainsworth, a student of Bowlby's, developed the theory further, describing patterns of secure and insecure attachment and pointing out the role of the parent to provide a secure base from which infants can explore and a safe haven to which they can return, thus emphasising the reciprocal relationship between autonomy and dependence (Ainsworth *et al.* 1978).

More recently Crittenden, Landini and Claussen (2001) suggested that insecure attachment patterns could be seen as self-protective responses to sub-optimal environments and that symptoms can be seen as adaptive strategies, rather than inevitably pathological responses.

Attachment theory suggests that depending upon the nature of their attachment, children develop different Internal Working Models (IWMs) which influence and predict their future adult relationships and in turn the attachment patterns towards their own children. Thus an understanding of parents' own attachment histories is vital when assessing their relationship with their own children.

In a residential setting the team needs to be aware of many attachment relationships, between parents and their children, between parents themselves and parents and their own families of origin. These will all influence how children and families relate to the team members. In addition, the attachment styles of the staff will be evident in their clinical work.

Patterns of attachment

Many of the children who use inpatient services have significant attachment problems. Mary Ainsworth and colleagues (1978) have divided insecure attachment patterns into two different categories: avoidant attachment and ambivalent/resistant attachment. Mary Main, another researcher in this area, added a further category of disorganised attachment (Main and Solomon 1986).

Children with *avoidant attachment* develop patterns of behaviour to control their closeness to carers who are consistently rejecting or overly intrusive. This may be expressed by becoming withdrawn or passive, with little display of emotional distress. These children are likely to develop an IWM of having trust in themselves but distrust towards other people. As adults they may be overly self-contained and struggle to maintain healthy intimate adult relationships. It is possible to see this pattern in some of David's behaviours (described on p.32 and p.143) or Ben's aggressive play (described on pp.73–75).

Ambivalent/resistant patterns of behaviour are characterised by intense emotional distress, for example, becoming demanding, oppositional or clingy. This pattern is thought to arise when carers are inconsistent in their care, so that at times the parent is available and emotionally responsive and at other times unavailable or rejecting. This is often seen in children whose parents have a relapsing mental illness or who intermittently misuse alcohol or other mind-altering substances. These children display extreme emotional distress and resistance to being comforted or nurtured. Their intense distress can be seen as a means of trying to maintain or regain a connection with their parents. Their IWM is one of needing others to contain their negative emotions, and fear of abandonment. This pattern of attachment in childhood can emerge in adulthood as emotional lability and dramatic behaviour that is used to manipulate family and friends.

When parents or carers frighten children or are themselves in a constant state of fear, children's behaviour becomes *disorganised*, because the carer is both the source of comfort as well as a source of distress. In a toddler this is seen as unpredictable behaviour that lacks a coherent strategy. Children may, over time, become self-reliant and controlling as a way of solving their dilemma. Their IWM might be of having a sense of power but also one of fear. Adults with this psychological make-up may become either abusers or recurrent victims of abuse.

In terms of attachment theory, a residential unit can be said to provide a safe and secure environment for children and their parents to relax and also for parents to be able to reflect or explore new ideas. The staff can help parents and children to negotiate negative emotions. Other parenting interventions, such as Mellow Parenting or Watch, Wait and Wonder (WWW), which are described later, will encourage parents to become more attuned to or sensitive to their children's emotional needs. As parents increase their attunement, they can begin to respond more appropriately to their children's attachment needs and with increased reciprocity (Howe *et al.* 1999).

In order to consider all these aspects referred to above, one has to consider:

- the environment and staff within it, providing a nurturing environment for both parents and children that enables therapeutic work to occur

- the parents attending the unit where one might be both assessing and/or aiming to enhance their nurturing skills, in regard to their children

- the organisation providing a nurturing or supportive environment for staff.

A nurturing environment

As stated above, nurturing is a very broad concept and therefore the ways in which a residential unit provides an environment that might be described as nurturing are numerous. This might range from the warm drinks offered to families entering the unit for the first time, to the non-judgemental approach inherent in all interactions with children and families, or to providing comfortable spaces, open communication and ensuring families are truly listened to.

This section illustrates how a nurturing environment has been created at the Croft unit. Other settings will naturally have their own local adaptations dependent on the client group they serve and the context and culture within which they operate.

At the Croft there is a parents' support group once a week; this usually entails a trip off the unit to a local coffee shop where parents and staff can sit comfortably in a non-institutional setting to chat. For many parents this will be the first time they have had such a social outing for months, if not years, as their lives have been consumed by caring for their children or managing their own difficulties. Many parents talk about becoming socially anxious in group settings after years of being virtually housebound, so being offered such a social event can be both challenging but also liberating.

Another aspect of nurturing can be giving parents an opportunity to play with art and craft materials or make music or join in playful activities with their children. This provides opportunities which many parents have lacked in their own impoverished childhood. Thus staff might suggest fun activities or games for parents to do with their children such as spotting rabbits in the wider grounds surrounding the Croft, or putting on a puppet show for other parents and staff, or a shared art activity. Children love the 'Croft joke fairy' who leaves a joke under their bedroom door whilst they are asleep if they managed their agreed bedtime routine. Some parents talk about a sense of achievement or just pure enjoyment after such fun activities, but others initially feel a sense of loss and maybe even depression as they realise what they lacked themselves as children.

Staff need to be sensitive or attuned to parental mood, making a cup of tea and offering to chat when needed, or giving parents space and not imposing demands. Being available to parents when needed and generally respectful of the parents' perspectives all contributes to creating an environment where parents feel valued and heard.

Staff also work hard, alongside parents, to create a nurturing atmosphere for the children. At the beginning of a family's stay it may well be staff members creating fun for the children but as the admission progresses, parents' confidence in their ability to engage positively with their child increases, they take over more and more of these activities and the staff can step back.

The programmes devised for school holiday periods are full of enjoyable activities that parents can participate in with their children, such as visits to the local park, bouncy castle, a trip to the seaside, and so on. Then, in ways like those described above with parents, staff aim to model the attunement and sensitivity to children's emotional states and moods for the parents to pick up and copy. Wherever possible this is done without taking over the parental role, but working alongside the parent and being available to step in as the need arises.

Role of non-clinical staff

Other key staff members who can help families feel comfortable and nurtured on the unit are the administration staff and the housekeeper.

Within large inpatient multi-disciplinary teams there is a very important role for support staff. They often have the most face-to-face contact with parents and they can provide a more informal style of support. They are often mature people with wide life experience who may have worked on the unit for several years and are able to provide a secure base for some parents. Those parents who have neglectful or abusive childhoods may experience authority figures as critical and frightening – so they may find themselves more able to speak to a non-clinical member of staff who they find less threatening than someone higher in the team hierarchy.

This relationship might start as fairly innocuous discussions with the housekeeper around their feelings of inadequacy about cooking, but may extend over time to disclosing very sensitive information, which they have not discussed with the rest of the team. Support staff often find themselves cast in the role of grandmother or aunt, both by children and adults. It is easy for staff in this position to find themselves under pressure to act as a surrogate family member, and for this reason and others it is essential that these team members have the same access to appropriate training, support and supervision as the clinical team. They must also follow the team protocols on sharing information where necessary, and be open with parents about the boundaries around confidentiality.

The housekeeper also provides a non-critical stance through working alongside parents, helping them plan healthy meals or to think about budgeting. Children make their request to the housekeeper for lunchtime sandwiches and she can create inexpensive nutritional meals which can be enjoyed on the unit and then copied by families at home. When a child leaves the unit a lunchtime party is held to celebrate, and the housekeeper will work with the parents to choose or make a special cake and make sure that the child's favourite foods are included. In all these roles the housekeeper can be thought of as providing a positive parenting or nurturing experience for parents.

> Patrick was in his fifth week at the Croft. There had been some discussion about extending his admission. Until this point Patrick's mother's emotional state had remained reasonably stable, with a combination of considerable support from unit staff and careful monitoring of her medication by her local adult mental services. However, at this point in the admission, she had begun to deal with some very difficult issues from her own past. She was also facing the concerns being voiced by social services about her lack of ability to meet Patrick's emotional needs. Staff were also increasingly worried that she was becoming overwhelmed and was at risk of becoming mentally unwell.
>
> During the same week Patrick's stepfather talked to a male member of staff about his own ill health and his fears for his wife. This was discussed at the weekly ward round and it was decided

that the team should offer Diane a few days off the unit to give her an opportunity to relax and look after her own emotional needs. It was also agreed that Patrick's stepfather would stay with him for a couple of days but then have time at home with his wife in order for them to have some time together as a couple. Patrick's parents and his key worker talked to him about this plan; they presented it as an opportunity for Patrick to be independent and to have time on the unit choosing his own activities. One of his key workers knew that he loved baking and he chose some recipes he would like to try. With some help from the housekeeper he cooked his own pizza for dinner. Later, as he was decorating biscuits, he talked to her about how much he missed his mum and how worried he was that she might have to go back to hospital.

The next day Patrick was able to provide some of the staff team with an array of decorated biscuits, for which he received accolades from everyone, which in its small way helped build his self-esteem. When Patrick's parents returned to the unit he excitedly told them about all the activities he had been doing and gave them their own biscuits decorated with the words 'I Love Mum' and 'I Love Dad'.

Enhancing parental nurturing skills

In addition to maintaining a supportive and nurturing environment using the framework and techniques described in the previous section, specific groups and therapies are used to stimulate nurturing experiences and skills; these include the Mellow Parenting programme, which will be described in the next chapter, the WWW approach and dyadic music and play sessions.

Infant mental health

Infant mental health is the developing capacity of the child from birth to three to experience, regulate and express emotions, to form close secure interpersonal relationships and to explore the environment and learn (Sameroff, McDonough and Rosenblum 2004). At the Croft, as in other child mental health services, a guiding principle is that positive infant mental health is essential to healthy social and emotional development. The interaction between parent and infant is the context in which emotional regulation evolves. According to Tronnick (1989), the mutual regulation model is dependent on both the child's capacity to control his homeostatic, affective and behavioural states and the caregiver's capacity to attune to the child's emotional state and facilitate the child's ability to self-regulate. The infant can only thrive through the support and responsive interactions of the primary caregiver.

When children have not been able to build these templates for self-soothing, they may develop disorders of impulse control. Cairns (2004) suggested that children with attachment disorders will show challenging behaviour due to deficits in their ability to manage their own impulses, and that this can lead on to a lack of moral accountability in adolescence and beyond. This ability to regulate negative emotions and to develop adaptive coping skills has also been shown to be important in protecting young people against the onset of depression in adolescence (Goodyer 2001). So attachment disorders and concomitant emotional dysregulation are likely to be significant contributors to both externalising and internalising disorders in later life.

Schore (2001) highlighted the importance of attachment status on the development of the neurobiological structure of the infant brain. During the first year of life the brain develops rapidly and the right hemisphere is central in moderating the child's stress response; in this manner the attachment relationship facilitates the expansion of the child's coping capacities and is a resilience factor for optimal development over later stages of the life cycle.

Stern (2004) emphasises the necessity in these situations to be mindful, when working with disadvantaged populations, that they have been frequently blamed, criticised and invalidated. As stated above, it was important to avoid becoming the critical parent and rather to use psychologically sensitive approaches to try to stimulate a change in the relationship between child and parent.

Watch, Wait and Wonder (WWW)

Watch, Wait and Wonder (WWW) is a therapeutic approach to attachment problems described by Muir, Lojkasek and Cohen (1999). A modified version of this is used at the Croft to help nurture the relationship between the child and the parent. It can be used with infants from around four months to children of nine years of age. Cohen (cited in *Muir et al.* 1999) suggests that WWW is indicated if there is a relationship problem, for example, attachment problems in conjunction with a parent saying she does not understand, is not bonded with and/or does not know how to play with her child.

WWW is a child-led psychotherapeutic approach. It encourages parents to observe and appreciate their child's spontaneous activity during free play to enhance maternal sensitivity and responsiveness. With enhanced parental acceptance come improvements in the child's sense of self and self-efficacy, emotion regulation and the child–parent attachment relationship. The approach provides space for the infant/child and parent to work through developmental and relational struggles through play. Also central to the process is engaging the parent to be reflective about the child's inner world of feelings, thoughts and desires, through which the parent recognises the separate self of the infant and gains an understanding of her own emotional responses to her child. WWW does not aim to teach parenting skills; rather parents are told that they and their child will discover ways of relating to each other. This method can reinforce competence and enjoyment in mothering.

The play session runs for approximately 20 to 30 minutes and during it the mother and the therapist both watch the child play, letting the child direct his play and only stepping in to support the play when necessary. The therapist encourages the parent to observe and think about what is happening for the child. In this way the mother is enabled to become more knowledgeable about her child and to reflect on her child's inner world, in other words, to develop a reflective capacity. The therapist sits beside the parent during the play and shares the experience but does not intrude. At the end of the session the parent is asked about the observations of her child's play and any difficulties she may have observed. In the discussion that follows, the therapist helps the parent to bring up any feelings of discomfort she may have had.

These sessions are offered weekly throughout the admission. This approach has much in common with the Mellow Parenting video approach described in Chapter 5, and in a similar vein provides another way to nurture parents, and encourage their growth and understanding of their child's difficulties. It also contributes to the overall assessment, giving further valuable insights into the nature of the relationship difficulties in the context of a nurturing environment.

Ben and Emma were referred to the Croft by Ben's social worker for an assessment of Emma's parenting capacity. Emma was a single mum of 21 and Ben was 18 months old.

Emma's own background was very troubled – when she was four her own mother had committed suicide and subsequently she and her siblings had been neglected by their father. Emma had been sexually abused by her older brother from the age of seven. As a teenager she had suffered bouts of depression and had repeatedly cut herself. She had misused alcohol for a while and tried a number of different illegal drugs. She had a series of boyfriends with whom she had stormy, sometimes violent, relationships. Previous mental health assessments had indicated that Emma had a personality disorder and she had been prescribed antidepressants and antipsychotic medication for her mood swings and anxiety and had regular contact with a community psychiatric nurse.

Emma had been ambivalent about her pregnancy and she had not had any prenatal care. She had been identified as having difficulties in coping on the postnatal ward after the birth and social services had become involved. Ben was placed on the 'at risk' register and Emma had regular visits from social workers, family support workers and her health visitor nurse. Emma had been honest with her health visitor that she felt unable to love Ben and was finding it increasingly difficult to provide for even his basic needs. She was struggling to manage his demands. Ben had no structure or routines in his life, and social services had put in a package of care but there had been little change for him. There were accounts of him not being supervised, Emma's drug misuse was becoming more evident and she was becoming more isolated as she refused to engage Ben in community activities.

Emotionally she appeared unable to provide Ben with consistency of care to begin to provide him with attachment security. Ben was experiencing unpredictable mothering and there were concerns that he was developing ambivalent, preoccupied behaviours, becoming whiny, clingy and having temper tantrums in an attempt to make a connection with his mother.

Over the eight-week stay, several interventions were used for attachment-based work to help focus on enhancing Emma's sensitivity towards Ben. One of these was WWW.

Emma was initially shown the WWW DVD. This introduced the idea that Emma could just sit alongside Ben while he played without having to think of how to play with him, which was appealing to her. Emma admitted that she felt she lacked the imagination or the will to sit and play with Ben.

The playroom was set up with a few of the toys from the unit. Staff had noted that Ben liked to play with building blocks, cars and his tiger.

Initially staff asked Emma to sit and observe without taking over the activity so that Ben led the play. Initially Ben went over to the building bricks, looked at his mum and then began to bang the brick with increasing aggression, looking over to Emma for a response.

When Emma had observed Ben for a while, staff asked her what her thoughts were and what the experience of observing Ben was like. The aim of this was to increase Emma's observational skills, to allow explorations of Ben's and Emma's experiences and to facilitate her reflective capacities.

Emma was at first puzzled by the question, but after some moments replied 'Pretty aggressive. I was thinking he might come over and hit me.' This discussion time with the staff provided an opportunity for Emma to think about Ben as she struggled to make sense of what Ben's play meant to her and led her to say she was 'rubbish' at being a mother. Staff had to try hard to encourage Emma to be interested in Ben rather than talk about her own distress. Ben immediately noticed this and came over to his mum, putting out his arms to be picked up. Emma said she found it too difficult to cuddle him. This encounter was to be repeated; it was painful for staff to observe this but it was further evidence that this was a very concerning case. Ben was left feeling distressed that his mother showed no inclination to be interested in him and nor was she available to him.

Ben would have felt rejected, abandoned by his mother who was unable to hold him in mind and was too preoccupied with her own difficulties to be able to be sensitive to his needs. Staff had to intervene to allay Ben's distress.

This pattern seemed pervasive; staff were often observing Emma's lack of response to Ben's demands. She appeared unable to interpret his emotions, particularly if he became distressed and angry. Staff were concerned that Emma could not soothe Ben when he was upset and sometimes her attempts to do so only led to him becoming more unhappy. Ben's rapid emotional swings seemed to be most prominent when he was with his mother. When he was playing with a staff member his moods seemed much more stable. Emma was often irritable and she would often hand Ben over to a member of staff if she could not settle him straight away.

Arising from these particular observations some initial feedback was given in a measured and sensitive way to Emma that staff were becoming increasingly concerned for Ben's wellbeing.

Nurturing staff

Looking after staff is an essential element for the smooth running of any organisation. Whilst patient care and safety is paramount, staff also need to be physically and emotionally robust to provide optimum care. The organisation must take measures to minimise harm to staff and seek to support their emotional health as well. This is particularly important in mental health services where staff are exposed to high levels of emotional distress and physical threat. This provision of a nurturing environment for staff will include providing adequate staffing, training, regular appraisal and supervision, debriefing and support groups. Underpinning this will be the quality of relationships between all staff.

As in the parenting process, this nurturing of staff has components that include not only the containing or holding aspects emphasised in the previous chapter, but also the more nurturing elements. To avoid duplication, supervision and support structures are discussed here.

Clinical supervision

Definitions

Much has been written about the clinical supervision process and whilst authors may differ in their definitions there appears to be a casual consensus within counselling and clinical psychology disciplines to support the definition provided by Bernard and Goodyear (2004). They described supervision as:

> an intervention provided by a more senior member of a profession to a more junior member or members of that same profession. This relationship is evaluative, extends over time, and has the simultaneousness purposes of enhancing

the professional functioning of the more junior person(s), monitoring the quality of professional services offered to the clients, she, he, or they see, and serving as a gatekeeper for those who are to enter the particular profession. (p.8)

The NHS Management Executive (1993, p.3) defined supervision as 'a formal process of professional support and learning which enables individual practitioners to develop knowledge and competence, assume responsibility for their own practice and enhance consumer protection and safety of care in complex situations'. It aims to identify solutions to problems, increase understanding of professional issues, improve standards of patient care, further develop skills and knowledge, and enhance practitioners' understanding of their own practice.

It is of note here that these definitions emphasise the monitoring or professional development aspects, although recognising the more supportive and perhaps nurturing components of supervision.

Within the unit, there are several supervision structures. These include the individual supervision provided regularly within the separate disciplines, group clinical supervision and the staff support group.

Individual supervision

Staff need opportunities in a trusting and safe atmosphere to discuss how they feel about patients, and to recognise resonances with their own personal circumstances, attachment relationships or past life events. Even staff with secure attachment representations may eventually become less nurturing if they are faced with constant rejection and hostility. For example, as in Patrick's case, if the child acts as though he does not need support and becomes very challenging, then it becomes more difficult for staff to feel empathy towards that child.

> Melissa was a nursing student who had come to the Croft for a six-week placement. After a couple of weeks on the unit she was asked to work alongside a senior nurse undertaking observations of Emma and Ben. The next day she rang in to say she was unwell. She came back to work a couple of days later and her nurse mentor arranged a supervision session. During the discussion Melissa talked

about her feelings of anxiety and anger when observing Emma and Ben. As the conversation proceeded Melissa talked about her own childhood. It emerged that she had been brought up by her single mother but had been left with her grandmother at the age of eight and had not seen her mother for the next ten years. The experience of working with Emma and Ben had brought back strong feelings of anger and abandonment from her past, leading to her becoming anxious and tearful.

Her mentor listened sympathetically to her account and reassured her that strong reactions to families were common. She suggested that she seek appropriate counselling and signposted her to a local service. It was agreed that Melissa would complete her placement but work mainly with the older children on the unit. The mentor spoke with Melissa's university supervisor to alert her to Melissa's difficulties so that consideration could be given to subsequent placements and so that she could get useful advice about her future career options.

Group clinical supervision

The group clinical supervision is held weekly and is facilitated by senior members of the multi-disciplinary team. The team will focus on a family chosen because they present a particularly worrying issue. The senior clinicians will help the team make a formulation (Carr 2006) of the issue. By integrating various branches of psychological theory, a formulation attempts to summarise a client or family's problems in terms of how they arose and what may currently be maintaining the difficulties. These explanatory ideas lead to working hypotheses, which are then used to suggest appropriate further assessments or interventions. A formulation can also be described as a means of translating theory to practice in clinical work. The ability to make intellectual sense of distressing and disturbed situations also creates a sense of coherence and confidence and increases staff emotional availability (Howe *et al.* 1999). Considering all the influences on a situation also helps team members to retain an overview of the issue and to avoid overly polarised viewpoints. An important part of this process is the acknowledgement that staff will have strong emotional responses to patients, especially those who have close direct contact with the children and their parents. For this reason it is very important to understand those psychodynamic processes of transferential and counter-transferential relationships and projections in order to respond positively to situations rather than reacting against them (Rolf 2001). This is discussed further in the section below on the externally facilitated staff support group.

The staff support group

At the Croft there is a group for the staff that meets weekly on a Friday afternoon, with an external facilitator, after the families have gone home for the weekend. For obvious reasons what follows does not include discussion of any of this particular group's processes or material, but it affords the chance to look more generally at some of the opportunities such a group might offer to a staff team and to consider the place of such groups in psychiatric settings.

Working in mental health settings is demanding. Staff in all professional areas are confronted constantly with the mental pain and psychological disturbance that have brought their patients into hospital; in a children's service of the kind that is offered by the Croft, they also have particularly high levels of contact with patients' parents and wider families, who may themselves be very distressed. Sustaining one's professional existence within such a complex and emotionally charged framework can be painful and exhausting, not simply because of the day-to-day busyness of things, but above all because of the powerful currents of projection and splitting that are active all the time outside the sphere of ordinary conscious communication or perception.

In the language of attachment theory, as referred to above, the Croft seeks to offer a secure base (Holmes 2002) within which patients and their families can find a place to address their difficulties, and which provides, through the staff's practice, containment, mature thought and consistent support. When staff feel overwhelmed by painful experiences and feelings, they may try to free themselves from them through denial, minimising their importance, holding others or the system responsible for everything, acting out, or simply assuming that there is nothing to be done. Whatever the nature of such a defensive response, it makes the possibility of active thought and of seeking to understand experience impossible, so although it may provide an attempted short-term fix to the pain of anxiety or other distress, it holds no prospect of more far-reaching change. On the other hand, a well-functioning staff team can offer two important things. First, they may provide the possibility of some attuned and active containment of feelings which makes it possible for those in distress, instead of turning away from a difficult experience, to face it more boldly, accept their own part in it and allow their capacity for creative engagement with difficulties to come into play. Second, simply in the nature of their dealings with one another and with families, the staff may model some healthier, more flexible way of being together which depends less on resorting to old assumptions and is more able to allow room for enquiry and for thinking together.

Staff members are human beings too, and are as subject to stress and anxiety (and ultimately unhelpful attempts to avoid them) as anyone else. It seems natural then, to ask what resources staff may need in order to enable them both to be as emotionally available as possible to patients and to manage their own experience. Bowlby's familiar proposal of the secure base needed by everyone in childhood is of an adult attachment figure to whom it is possible to turn for protection, security and nourishment (Bowlby 1998). A secure attachment figure is not someone who is there all the time, but rather someone whose continuing availability allows children to feel able to go off and explore, both physically and emotionally, with the sure knowledge that they can return to the security of their attachment figure when they need to, and that that person will be interested in their experience and help them to make sense of it. Without that certainty, they are much less likely to be adventurous or to seek new encounters. In adult life the needs for security may change in their nature but are no less important.

In mental health services a staff group needs to be able to offer its members a space in which they can really attend to one another, think together about their experience and explore feelings, including those of difference or disagreement, without resorting to some sort of collusive denial of difficulty. These are, after all, fundamental things that staff in a good clinical environment will seek to offer patients; if staff are to be able to do that, however, they need those things just as much to be available to them as well, and the secure base of a staff group may be one such resource.

Difficult, frustrating or conflicted exchanges with patients may leave staff members with feelings of their own that are unwelcome and hard to bear. That can make the task of containment – of somehow managing to hold on to the feelings projected by the patient, thinking about them and offering them back to the patient in a form that makes them more tolerable and a potential starting point for change – seem burdensome and perhaps impossible. If the feelings that arise within staff cannot be faced, or their importance or existence is denied, there is a risk of acting on these feelings unconsciously in ways that are potentially harmful both to patients and to working relationships with colleagues; if staff can allow themselves to voice these feelings and seek to understand them, such discussion may enormously enrich their practice.

The notion of a staff group as a team, with its associated implications of collaboration, mutual understanding and shared responsibility, is something well established in a wide range of health care settings. But to function smoothly and effectively in that way is not always easy, especially in circumstances where levels of psychological and emotional strain may be high. To be called a team is no guarantee of being able consistently to act as one. For that to become more possible, individual members need to be more aware of their own and others' feelings and the part they play, consciously and unconsciously, in their interactions with one another and with their patients. There is the risk instead of a resort to what Speck (1994) has called 'chronic niceness', through which the group may seek to split off negative feelings about themselves, each other or their patients and direct them towards patients' relatives, other professionals, or some outside and unreachable force (the management, the NHS as a whole, the government, and so on), whilst maintaining a façade of comfortable supposed mutual understanding and acceptance.

When staff members can become aware, however, that they are not alone in their feelings, the group can be more available as a container and through that can, as a whole, better understand its own functioning, and so operate together in a more integrated way. Such a group is not one in which there is no disagreement, envy or other difficulties, but rather one in which those things can be acknowledged and worked through when they arise without the fear that doing so will risk some sort of breakdown of working relationships. It is also a place where the realities of differences between group members (of profession, age, experience, status, level of training) may be recognised, and their impact on team relationships considered. All this is far from easy, but if team members do not have the opportunity to consider together the impact upon themselves, individually and collectively, of their encounters with patients and with one another, then difficult feelings may become even more deeply buried and ultimately create greater disturbance: 'Difficult emotions that remain unconscious may block clear thinking' (Winship 1995, p.231).

There is a growing body of outcome research in mental health which suggests that patients who are cared for by teams who routinely meet as a group in this way will have better outcomes than those who are not. There are also indications that teams who attend a staff group of this kind have lower levels of sickness and staff turnover (Haigh 2000).

For such a group to work usefully together there are some basic practical necessities. The group needs a comfortable meeting room, a regular and agreed time (normally one hour every week), and an understanding that the session will not be interrupted except in the case of emergency. Staff members are asked to make attendance at the group a priority. Staff unable to attend should send a message to the group. There will be an agreement that events in the group will not be discussed outside it without the permission of those concerned and that the facilitator will share that commitment to confidentiality. All of these things may contribute not just to the smooth practical running of the group, but to a shared sense of ownership of it and of its ongoing life.

A facilitator who has no other connection with the staff group or their patients is potentially able to think with independence about what is taking place, to be impartial and to respond without judgement. He seeks to draw attention to what may be going on or to events that appear to be being ignored, and to wonder about what may not be being said. That in turn may enable the group to pursue more readily its tasks of finding greater understanding and appreciation between members and of becoming able to let the group become a useful space for thought and for recognition of differences. A group that is moving towards these things in a spirit of openness is more likely to find communication and working relations between members strengthened, with corresponding benefits for the unit as a whole and the patients whom it serves.

On Friday afternoon, the team met as usual. As often happened the group took some time to warm up and the opening discussion was general and focused on events and incidents not obviously related to the Croft. There was a fair bit of laughter as jokes were shared. A nurse commented that another colleague looked 'knackered', to which she replied curtly that it had been a hard week, but did not expand. The conversation again took off in another direction, again not obviously related to work issues. There was a period of silence, finally broken by the facilitator who gently suggested that something was being avoided. This was quickly followed by a senior member of the nursing team who started to speak about her concerns about Emma and whether the team would eventually be recommending that Ben should be taken into care. Another therapist said she had observed some really positive aspects to Emma's interactions with Ben in a therapy session and she felt that the team should remain open-minded. The consultant at this point expressed some feelings about how tough it felt, writing the reports which could be crucial in deciding the child's future. At this point, Jan, usually a quiet younger member of the nursing team, suddenly opened up and, close to tears, confessed that she felt very differently from most of her colleagues, and couldn't see how the team could even think about Emma losing Ben. Although she did not say so, most people in the room were aware that she had two small preschool children, one of whom was a very similar age to Ben.

Following this there was an extended discussion about Ben and Emma. The team, although it was not clear-cut, seemed to divide between the more junior nursing staff on the one hand, who felt that the team should remain hopeful about Emma's ability to parent Ben, and the senior members of the multi-disciplinary team who felt less optimistic about Ben's future with Emma. The facilitator commented quietly on this apparent divide. Another team member then commented on Jan's personal situation with her two small boys who she was struggling to leave at home to come to work. There was considerable sympathy and understanding expressed in the room for her situation. It also helped another member of staff to express her feelings about Emma and Ben and how distressing she had found the play session with them.

The session ended with the facilitator commenting that the dilemmas facing the team were emotionally very stressful and at times hard to articulate, but that despite the different views in the team, relationships could be maintained.

Summary

This chapter set out to describe the variety of ways that nurturing is available in the context of the Croft by creating a supportive environment, through direct work with children and parents themselves, and to support the staff team. Nurturing is a key ingredient in the therapeutic mix necessary to work with complex families and children. It works alongside the containment and structure of the programme to create a safe and secure environment.

It is important, however, that the environment does not become so nurturing that families become enmeshed or so dependent on the unit that they are unable to leave positively; the aim is, rather, to provide a springboard from which families can move forward positively with their lives.

All the issues described in this chapter will have relevance for other child and family-focused services but they are much more prominent in intensive or residential care settings. Lack of attention to these areas will put a service at risk of fragmentation and failure.

With containment, structure and nurturance in place, the family and the team can move on to use the therapeutic opportunities available to address problems and to find solutions. These specific therapeutic approaches are described in the following chapters but interwoven with them are frequent references to these fundamental concepts.

Chapter 5

Multi-Family Work

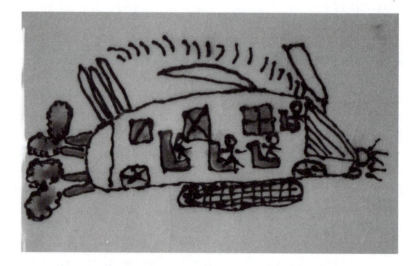

Andy remembered fun trips out with other families

Introduction

Most mental health inpatient facilities for children in the UK admit the child to the ward and invite families to attend the unit regularly for therapy sessions and to visit their child. Routinely admitting children with a parent or parents (and sometimes siblings) for all or most of the admission is therefore an unusual model. Obviously this approach allows the team to assess children within their family context, but it also creates a multi-family environment and this is an important aspect of the assessment and treatment model at the Croft Unit. The emphasis on family admissions was one of the founding principles of the Croft service, based on the principle that a fully holistic assessment of children with complex mental health problems can only be achieved if they are assessed within their family context, and that changes in both the individual and the family are usually necessary to achieve positive, sustainable, outcomes for these children.

Although this chapter focuses on the particular setting at the Croft Child and Family Unit, the majority of the principles discussed would apply in a wider range of settings, wherever a number of families come together in a group setting. This could include children's centres, schools and parent support groups.

Much of the multi-family work at the Croft happens informally, in the mornings and evenings, or during holiday periods when family activities are the focus of the programme. There are some more formal sessions, such as the Mellow Parenting groups and other groups during which parents and children participate together.

Multi-family group therapy (MFGT)

Over the last three decades, the therapeutic opportunities that a multi-family group setting offers have become increasingly evident to the unit team, and this has coincided with a burgeoning body of research supporting the value of a multi-family group approach to a range of disorders including schizophrenia and anorexia nervosa. The practice of multi-family group therapy (MFGT) with 'multi-problem families' in a day unit has been described by the Marlborough Family Service in London (Asen 2002).

MFGT combines the principles of group work and systemic family therapy and encompasses ideas from both psychodynamic and attachment theories. The strengths, skills and concerns of families are shared within the group so that parents and children become as important as the staff facilitators in generating change. In effect, families consult one another. The group context widens the range of ideas and experiences that families are working with, whilst enriching the quality of self-reflection.

Community living

In outpatient settings, families may meet other families informally in the waiting room, and parents or children may meet others through attending groups, but it is rare that whole families meet together for any extended period. Sharing day-to-day activities as well as more formal therapy sessions can be a particularly powerful experience, especially in the heightened emotional circumstances or 'pressure cooker effect' that most families find themselves in when their child is in crisis.

A further advantage of working with several families concurrently is that it dilutes the sense each family has of being 'the problem family', instead creating a community of families facing similar challenges. This shared experience reduces the families' fear that being observed by professionals whilst parenting their children will inevitably lead to being held wholly responsible for their children's problems (Croft 2004). Comments by parents during a qualitative study at the Croft (Rivington 2008) described how they found the camaraderie amongst parents to be a significant source of support and a welcome distraction to the emotional turmoil of their treatment. They also appreciated 'having an adult conversation and talking about life' (p.24).

Clinical experience would suggest that the majority of parents gain from the presence of other families in the unit. Their experience of social isolation and exclusion as a consequence of their child's difficult behaviour can be profound, and is frequently mentioned by parents. They talk about feeling judged and rejected by other parents in the school playground, and losing contact with friends and family. If their child is excluded from school they will then be further excluded from everyday social contact. Many parents have had to give up work due to their child's difficulties, and some parents avoid making intimate adult relationships because of the inevitable strain on such relationships due to their child's special needs.

Managing complex group dynamics

Whilst there are many beneficial aspects to community living there are also negative aspects to the experience, as anyone who has lived in shared accommodation will recall. A few parents (and children) become over-involved and over-identified with another family that may divert their energies from dealing with their own problems. Occasionally a child will make an alliance with another parent, undermining her relationship with her own parent. The powerful dynamics produced by such alliances can lead to splits within the resident group and these must be managed sensitively and proactively by the staff to avoid any parent or child feeling victimised or abused by others.

Sometimes personalities clash and families often have different values and cultural backgrounds. Families admitted to the Croft come from diverse socio-economic and cultural groups but this rarely appears to be a major issue, as parents discover more issues in common than not. The very experience of being admitted to a mental health unit, with all that entails, is itself a shared experience that binds families together.

If parents share similar traumatic backgrounds, one family's disclosure can resonate with another family's history, inadvertently exacerbating existing distress. However, more often families find that sharing similar experiences reduces their sense of isolation and guilt.

Group processes

There are many experiences arising out of group interactions that influence parents and families during their admission. These mirror the processes that have been described in the literature about adult psychotherapy groups (Yalom 1985) and milieu therapy. These concepts include:

- *Universality*: the sharing of experiences and feelings amongst group members and the recognition that these are human concerns can lead to a reduction in individuals' sense of isolation. It also validates their experiences, and raises their self-esteem. Many parents say that seeing their child within a group including other children with significant special needs helps them to feel less isolated and to be able to see their child's problems in a wider perspective. Families observe other parents and children and seek similarities or differences. Parents often perceive other parents to be in the 'same boat' as them, and identify common challenges.

- *Altruism*: the opportunity to help others in the group gives a novel experience of having something to offer to others, thus raising self-esteem and encouraging adaptive coping styles and improved interpersonal skills. Often parents talk about the importance of establishing friendships and the pleasure they get from helping other parents.

- *Instillation of hope*: a mixed group will have members at various stages of their treatment, and those who are at a later stage of their treatment can encourage newer members of the group that progress is possible. Since within the unit families are arriving weekly, the families who are approaching the end of the programme are often a great support to the new arrivals, reassuring them and helping them through the emotional turmoil of the first few days.

- *Imparting information*: group members can share pertinent information with each other, thus widening their experience and expertise about their disorders and problems. Parents constantly share information about their child's care and experiences that they have found helpful. They may get great emotional support from sharing similar concerns, or indeed receive a great deal of useful information or practical advice on common problems from other parents.

- *Imitative behaviour*: group members observe and imitate each other and the therapists, thus acquiring a wider repertoire of more adaptive behaviours. It is well known that first-hand experience is a key aspect of learning and change. The staff team are well aware that parents watch closely how they manage children on the unit and they therefore model positive parenting strategies. Parents frequently comment on the staff's way of managing their children and can be seen to incorporate some of their styles into their own repertoire.

  Less is known about the extent to which parents model behaviours to other parents in this type of setting. However, clinical experience would indicate that parents also report noting the way other parents manage their children and this can stimulate reflection on their own behaviour in a similar situation. For example, parents might comment on the amount of praise given by another parent to her child with positive outcomes or decide to reduce negative comments if they have seen another parent being very hostile. There is of course a risk that parents might copy less adaptive means of dealing with their children, but clinical experience suggests that this is a very rare occurrence and, if it does emerge as an issue, staff step in to discuss this with parents directly.

- *Cohesiveness*: humans are social animals and their personal development reflects the social group they live in. If the group is supportive, accepting and cohesive, then the individual will show positive social development. Some parents say that living at the unit has given them their first experience of a positive, nurturing social experience where they feel accepted and valued.

- *Catharsis*: telling one's story to a supportive and validating group leads to a sense of relief from sharing the emotional burden with others. Often during the first couple of weeks on the unit, parents will share their family story in great detail, not just in formal therapy sessions, but also in informal social settings. Sometimes they disclose information that they have never spoken of before. Whilst this can be a highly emotional experience, often parents report a huge sense of relief when their story is heard and accepted and does not lead to rejection.

Informal multi-family settings

Whilst living communally there are many times during which families find themselves together: cooking a meal, watching television or playing a game of Monopoly, for example. The mornings and evenings at the Croft are the times when family life is most closely mirrored. The combination of informality and the heightened anxieties and emotions that become exposed during these periods allows families to open up more to both staff and other parents. Often the particularly difficult moments are the 'must be done' routines of family life. Mealtimes, bathtimes, bedtimes and getting children ready for school in the morning are often key moments when parents are under pressure to complete basic routines. Children often sense this and have learnt that they can create maximum impact by resisting these routines.

As in most households, the kitchen is the hub of the unit. Often the most sensitive conversations happen as the kettle is boiling or the evening meal is being prepared.

Parents are encouraged to sit with their children at the beginning of the evening to plan their activities – often this is done in a multi-family setting as each family negotiates when they will be cooking or spending time in the art or music rooms.

Inevitably with three or four families sharing a small space, there will occasionally be clashes and conflicts; most of these are resolved as they arise, but over time the team have found it essential to have a formal multi-family meeting each week to discuss housekeeping issues. The nursing team facilitate this meeting and model problem-solving and compromise to enable the families to resolve any conflicts. It is here that differences between families, such as eating, dietary and hygiene habits, might get exposed – this can sometimes lead to strong emotive opinions. This group has a practical focus of sorting out day-to-day living arrangements but also encouraging parents and children to communicate about conflictual issues and to feel able to address issues such as which food to choose to buy and share, cleanliness, and so on. Again the staff model strategies for using a calm, problem-solving approach and some families will adopt this approach at home and call family meetings to tackle problems in everyday household routines.

> David and Patrick's mums, Sarah and Diane, had decided to cook a meal together. This joint activity was much planned and both women enjoyed shopping for the meal together as well as preparing it. Stacey (Nick's mum) was chatting to them as they cooked. Nick had been watching television quietly whilst the mums were cooking in the kitchen. When he went to ask his mum if he could have his electronic game, Stacey told him that he could not have it as computer games were not allowed at the unit.
>
> Nick became very angry and he started to swear and kick Stacey. She seemed powerless to stop him, so staff quickly intervened and asked her what she wanted to do. They all agreed that Nick's behaviour needed to be contained and that he needed to go to the time out room to calm down. The staff explained this to Nick and he reluctantly agreed to go, but half way along the corridor he started to kick the staff so they quickly escorted him to the soft room where he could let off steam safely.
>
> Angela (Arthur's mum) witnessed the incident and became anxious and worried about Nick. A discussion followed between all the mums about children's aggression and how to deal with it. Stacey was worried that Nick would be very angry with her

for agreeing that the staff could take him to time out. She was concerned that it was too harsh a consequence and said that at home she would have put up with his aggression or given in to his demands to avoid a scene. She added that it would be impossible to put in a consequence at home as she didn't have a safe space and couldn't imagine herself persuading him to go there. Angela commented that other children that she had met on the unit had been just as aggressive as Nick but had benefited from clear consequences following physical aggression. Although this comment didn't answer Stacey's main doubts, it did allow her to accept the staff intervention at that moment a little more easily.

No sooner had Nick calmed down, than Arthur began to become agitated, as he didn't want to go to bed. Angela had been watching the 1, 2, 3 Magic video (Phelan 2003) that afternoon with Sarah. The video had emphasised the need to show less emotional response to challenging behaviour as well as putting in clear consequences to different levels of difficult behaviour. While they watched this, Sarah had admitted that she recognised her own strong emotional responses to David's behaviour, and also that she'd noticed Angela doing the same. As a result, Angela felt particularly conscious of her need to remain calm. She took deep breaths and remained calmer than she might have done in the past as she reminded Arthur that he needed to settle down.

Arthur's parents had not mentioned a sleep problem in their initial assessment. 'In the overall scheme of things, it wasn't a major problem for us,' they told night staff. They were used to the fact that Arthur was falling asleep on the settee around 10.30 p.m. at night, waking again at 3.00 a.m. and spending the rest of the night in his parents' bed. It wasn't until Philippa's mum had made a passing comment about what a nuisance that must be that Arthur's parents began to think about using their stay as an opportunity to tackle this problem.

As it happened, Diane was also working on a sleep programme for Patrick, and they were able to observe the struggle she was having. At one level this made them all the more sceptical about ever tackling this successfully; at another they were astute enough to recognise that Patrick and Arthur were quite different children and that they might be more successful.

The night staff were on hand to encourage and support parents by ensuring a calming environment, quiet voices, dimmed lights, and so on, and using strategies that fitted with Arthur's particular individual characteristics. In the end, parents and staff in collaboration had agreed to use a chart involving Arthur's maps. Angela had also picked up that children at the Croft were sometimes rewarded in the morning by the 'Croft fairy' leaving a small picture or joke under their door if they had successfully achieved their pre-arranged goal, and Arthur seemed to love this. She found herself increasingly confident to leave Arthur alone in his bedroom while she had a bath, as other parents had offered to let her know if he woke up or demanded her presence.

Such interactions are the day-to-day experiences in a unit where families with complex children live together and share a short, intense period of their lives. Whilst these lived moments are difficult to describe in terms of therapeutic models, they certainly can be profound emotional experiences that may well have more impact than more formal therapy sessions.

Although on the whole it tends to be mothers who are resident with their children, fathers often visit in the evenings. Sometimes fathers can feel excluded from their child's treatment and involvement with services, but if they are able to spend time with their family in the evenings, the informal, family-orientated atmosphere can help fathers re-engage with the process and also with their child.

Arthur's father, Martin, had been a difficult person to get to know, and had initially spent any free time he had at the Croft working on his laptop. He stayed with Arthur for a couple of nights to give his wife a break, and during this short stay he started to talk to a male staff member about his work and his love of technology. Later the conversation moved on to his genuine concerns about his son and his future. The men discussed Arthur's great love of construction and how this could be used as an opportunity to spend positive time with him. The next evening Martin asked him if he would show him how to make some LEGO models. After an initial hesitation Arthur agreed and an hour later he and his father had made an impressive model of a crane.

Facilitated therapy groups

Mellow Parenting

The Mellow Parenting programme (Puckering 2004) was originally designed for families with a preschool child who had severe attachment and behavioural difficulties. In particular, it addressed those families who were faced with a constellation of social and interpersonal problems and who had been unable to access standard community interventions.

The approach puts a strong emphasis on the engagement process, nurturing parents and working directly with parents and children in a group setting. In these respects the programme fitted with the philosophy and practice of the unit.

Mellow Parenting is usually run as a 14-week programme during which families attend for a day each week. Each day starts with a workshop for parents to share their experiences. These sessions are structured by the group facilitators and there are worksheets to stimulate and guide discussion. The themes in these sessions are wide-ranging and include childhood experiences at home and school, early intimate relationships, childbirth and experiences as a parent. During these sessions the group facilitators provide good coffee and nice biscuits – not the usual institutional beverages and plain biscuits – to signal how much the parents are valued and to reflect a more social group experience.

There is also an emphasis on the staff becoming active participants in the discussion rather than just facilitating. Thus if the discussion was about early childhood experiences, the staff members would also share information about their childhood. This can be a new and challenging experience for some mental health professionals whose professional training often includes a strong belief that professional boundaries should be maintained and that personal experiences should not be shared with service users. Breaking down this boundary, and sharing information that the professional feels comfortable with, dramatically changes the group experience, and parents often comment on this difference very favourably. They say that the group feels less formal and they feel less judged. They also experience the staff members as more human and are therefore more likely to share information with them in a less inhibited way.

In order to adapt this programme to the unit residential setting, the team decided to revise an existing parent support group. The group had often had poor attendance and many parents had described the pressure to talk about problems in a group setting as uncomfortable and intimidating. The group leaders decided to move the group out of the unit and to hold it in a local coffee shop. This normalised the group and provided an ordinary social experience and good coffee. Taking the group into a community setting also changed the dynamic between parents and staff.

Although the parent group is usually predominately female, when fathers are resident, a male member of staff is part of the group to balance the gender ratio and to support the fathers in giving the male perspective on issues discussed in the group.

Having a positive experience in this group builds group cohesion and supports parents to tackle more demanding therapeutic sessions. Parents can also use this context to bring up issues that they are unhappy with in regard to their admission, such as a difficult interaction with a staff member or a disagreement with a fellow resident. As the senior nurse manager usually facilitates this group, she is able to hear how families are feeling about their admission, and to proactively identify any issues arising indicating problems with the service.

The staff facilitators also introduce topics for discussion, such as beliefs about what would constitute an ideal family, or attitudes to education or child discipline. The staff encourage a free-flowing, non-judgemental conversation. They avoid an expert position and become participants, not observers or assessors.

> The topic for the parental workshop was childhood experiences and what it meant to be a 'good mum'. The icebreaker activity was for each person to share the story of how their name was chosen by their parents – this caused much amusement. Then one of the staff facilitators started the conversation by describing her own mother, a very traditional woman who had become a widow at an early age. The staff member talked about how much she had admired her mother but found it difficult to confide in her because she didn't want to burden her further. Philippa's mum, Jane, picked up this theme and spoke about her own childhood. She had always felt very close to her mother, Sue, and rather afraid of her strict and rather distant father. She had always felt a great need to please

her mother, especially after her father had died. She talked about how dependent she had been on Sue's help to look after Philippa when her older daughter Clare was in hospital as a young child. Jane talked about how much she felt in her mother's debt. At this point Arthur's mum commented that perhaps Philippa's grandma had enjoyed looking after Philippa, as it might have made her feel wanted and needed. Philippa's mum nodded and sadly reflected that Philippa had been so close to Sue that when she was small she had often cried bitterly when her mum had picked her up from her grandmother's house.

Stacey chipped in and brusquely said 'Being a kid is rubbish – I would never want to go back.' Other mums disagreed and talked about happy memories from their childhoods but the staff facilitator turned to Stacey and asked her about what being a good mum meant to her. She looked a little tearful but managed to say: 'A good mum looks after her kids and notices if they are miserable.' Everyone was quiet for a few seconds and there was a palpable sense of sympathy for Stacey. Then Sarah said 'That's why we are all here – because we care about our kids.' Everyone nodded.

Parent–child activity sessions

In the Mellow Parenting programme, whilst the parents are in their group together the children are enjoying a nursery session nearby. The children and parents have lunch together and then enjoy a simple fun activity together. This might be decorating cookies or making Christmas cards. This activity session is videoed and, in the afternoon parent session, the group look at the video together. In the unit setting the children are in group sessions whilst the parents are meeting. Staff then take videos of the families when they are playing together in the evenings or during a parent–child activity group.

Video feedback

The unit has a tradition of videoing parents and children in play or music sessions and then reviewing the tapes with the parent to look at parent–child interactions and encourage more positive engagement. The Mellow Parenting approach also makes much use of videotaping children and parents together and then using them within the multi-family group sessions.

Short video clips are taken of each parent with their child. The clips might feature the family eating a meal together or painting a picture or playing a board game. The parent group then sit together and watch clips that they have chosen of themselves. The group leader encourages everyone to focus on the positive aspects of parent–child interaction to encourage, empower and raise parents' self-esteem. Watching a video also allows parents to take a step back from their face-to-face interactions with their child and to reflect on these interactions, both what the child is doing but also how their own behaviour and emotional tone are affecting the interaction.

The staff facilitator may pause the video from time to time and ask questions such as 'What were you thinking about at this point?' or 'How do you think [child] is feeling now?' The ability to reflect on one's own role in an interaction is vital when trying to improve chronically negative relational patterns. Usually when asked about their child's problems, parents will be very clear about the child's negative behaviour, but they are often less consciously aware of how their own behaviour might have triggered or amplified a negative interaction.

After years of coping with severe behavioural problems in their children, parents often have very low confidence in their own parenting skills. Seeing video evidence of their child's enjoyment when playing with them, or even just their child washing her hands when asked, can be a very powerful experience. Parents are usually very generous in their praise of their fellow group members and hearing positive comments from a peer is often much more influential than hearing the same comment from a professional. Everyone is encouraged to be very specific in their comments, for example, a parent might say that she noticed how a parent got down to the child's level and showed interest in her child's activity in a non-verbal way. In other circumstances this brief interaction would have gone unnoticed but by highlighting it in this group, it serves both to improve that parent's sense of competence and also to show a behaviour worth emulating. The process itself has the added advantage of improving each person's observation skills. Often children want to see the video footage as well, and having a subsequent session with the child and parent together can also be very beneficial.

Whilst the focus of the video session is to catch positive interactions, it often leads on to a discussion about how to manage challenging behaviours as these may appear in footage alongside the positive material. Staff facilitators take an active role, alongside the parents, in brainstorming about positive ways of coping with challenging behaviour and encouraging pro-social behaviour, and this aspect of the group can consolidate conversations that occur in a parallel behaviour management group.

> The video feedback group started with all the parents anxiously giggling and saying how much they hated watching themselves on video. Angela said that she was used to it now after so many weeks and that she really enjoyed seeing video footage of Arthur enjoying various activities. The video clips this week had been taken during a trip to a local park to feed the ducks. The facilitator asked if anyone would like to pick a clip of themselves with their child. Diane said she would like to pick a clip this week. This surprised the facilitator as she had previously needed a lot of encouragement to show clips. The clip showed Diane and Patrick feeding bread to the ducks and then Diane pushing Patrick on a swing. At the end of the clip Patrick suddenly jumped off the swing and started running away from the playground, closely followed by Diane and a member of staff. They caught up with him and brought him back to the playground.
>
> As the clip was shown there were lots of positive comments from the mums about Diane and her interactions with Patrick. Someone mentioned how much she was smiling and how Patrick watched her expressions so closely. Sarah pointed out a moment when Patrick reached up to hold Diane's hand. Diane's eyes filled with tears at that point. She said it reminded her of how Patrick had been as a little toddler and how she wished he was like that more often.
>
> The group talked about how worrying it was when Patrick ran off – the staff facilitator asked Diane what she thought had triggered off that reaction. Diane said that sometimes when things were going well Patrick seemed to get panicky and do something to spoil it. The staff facilitator suggested that maybe Patrick wasn't confident that positive times could last – Diane thought about this and agreed that there had been a lot of uncertainty in his life.

Behaviour management group

A key therapeutic approach with a considerable evidence base in childhood is behaviour therapy. This therapeutic model underpins most parenting skills work and forms the bedrock to the management of challenging behaviour in children with a diverse range of difficulties. The behaviour management group for parents provides a structured setting for discussing behavioural issues and often picks up on issues that have been raised in other settings.

A challenge for this group, alongside the diversity of problems that parents are facing, is that it operates as an open group so that new parents are joining the group each week. Therefore the purpose and structure of the group needs to be constantly restated. However, a benefit of the open group is that parents who are in the latter stages of their admission can encourage newer residents and empathise with their understandable anxieties. This support from graduating parents appears to be an important factor in motivating parents to persist with the group, even if they feel very ambivalent initially.

Many parents who have been involved with child mental health services over an extended period have often had a great deal of input under the title of 'Behaviour Management'. For them, the emphasis on themselves as parents and instructions to alter their parenting style may have been frustrating. They may have interpreted this as an implication that all of their child's problems are caused by failures in their parenting. If they have attended parenting groups in the community they often say that the groups are dealing with much less severe behavioural problems than those shown by their children. The approach within the unit is to accept that parents are doing their best, that their children are not 'ordinary' and that they therefore need extra-ordinary parenting. With this as a premise, parents are much more willing to consider behavioural approaches to moderating their child's extreme behaviours.

The group facilitators create a culture within the group that validates experience and welcomes ideas. The focus is on participation, and whilst staff have professional expertise and experience of working with a wide range of children, it is stated that staff do not have all the answers and that parents hold the most rich and wide-ranging information about their own children. One way to illustrate this is by asking the parents the ages of all their children and then calculating the total years of parenting experience that the group collectively have. This immediately gives parents a sense that they are genuinely respected for the experience they bring to the group. It is not unusual for the total years of parenting in the room (including staff's personal experience) to add up to more than a century, giving everyone pause for thought.

In this group a problem-solving model is used. The rationale for this is that for parents who have had considerable previous input, it is likely that a didactic approach would be repeating previously futile work. Having experienced frustration and failure in groups before, parents may not be beyond the contemplative or even pre-contemplative stage of change (Prochaska, DiClemente and Norcross 1992). Some of the challenge therefore is dealing with parental resistance, and fostering a readiness to consider change (Miller and Rollnick 2002).

The other advantage of the problem-solving model is that it allows for a broader perspective, to include family and systemic models rather than a narrower focus on purely behavioural techniques. The group focuses on one child each week and considers the behaviour that the parent is most worried about in detail. The behaviour is carefully defined and broken down into its constituent parts and the factors that might be triggering or maintaining the behaviour are brainstormed. Once this is done then the group comes up with a range of suggestions about how the behaviour could be reduced. Parents then choose an idea to try during the following week and they report back on the outcome of their efforts at the beginning of the next group. The idea can then be adjusted if necessary. The emphasis is on achieving small successes.

> As it was Stacey's first week she was happy to take a back seat and find out more about how the behaviour management group ran. It was Arthur's tenth week and Angela had been an enthusiastic and regular group member. She was able to report that she'd been working on Arthur's bedtime routine. Progress had been slow over the first few weeks of their stay, but she was able to report considerable improvement over the previous week. She had tried an idea, suggested by one of the nurses, to create a bedtime map with pictures of some of his favourite landmarks on it, and to suggest that Arthur could move along the map (one street per night if he

remained in his room at bedtime). If he completed the map over a week he could then choose a treat. Angela and his key worker discussed the plan with Arthur and he had helped to make the map. Each morning he had been keen to draw his path along each street and his mum reported that whilst Arthur was still quite wakeful at night he was much more amenable to going into his bedroom and settling into bed.

The group were very positive and admiring of her efforts and Arthur's progress and talked about why this approach had worked when previous reward charts had not. In particular other parents were able to point out that they'd noticed how much more confident Angela had become, and that her way of talking to Arthur had become clearer and more authoritative. She was very pleased with this feedback. The conversation then moved on to discuss why it might sometimes be worth revisiting strategies that had not been successful in the past.

Patrick's mum, Diane, had previously been rather scathing of and reluctant to attend the group. However, this week, to the facilitators' surprise, she appeared willing for the first time to put Patrick's problem forward for the group to look at. She'd struck up a friendship with David's mum, and her friend's presence in the group helped to give her the confidence to be in the spotlight. However, she was still rather anxious as she started out, telling the group straight away that she had tried everything her social workers had suggested, to no effect. Her unsaid message seemed to be that it would be highly unlikely that anyone at the unit could possibly find any solution to her difficulties. The facilitators listened attentively and remained neutral, agreeing that her problems, like everyone else's in the group, were very complex. However, as she started to talk about her worries about Patrick she became very thoughtful and was able to think of times when he had been able to manage, as well as the times that his behaviour felt out of control.

Diane chose to focus on Patrick's non-compliance. Despite this being a rather broad set of behaviours, the group was able to ask her clarifying questions about how often this was a problem and in what sort of situations he was most likely to disobey her.

Using a basic ABC approach of antecedents, behaviours and consequences, Diane was unable to identify any pattern to his behaviour, but was able to describe in great detail how he'd scream and throw things at her in order to get his own way. The group asked about whether there were any times that he did not show such behaviour, and despite her initial reluctance to admit any exceptions, Diane did say that he appeared to behave better when he was on his own with either her or his stepfather. She also recalled one year in school when his behaviour had been better, which she attributed to Patrick responding well to a teacher whose teaching style was very firm and structured.

She then went on to say that his behaviour had always been difficult but had worsened after her admission to a psychiatric hospital following an overdose when she was very depressed. She told the group that whilst she had been in hospital her ex-boyfriend had looked after Patrick and may have sexually abused him. The group responded to this self-revelation with considerable sympathy. Stacey was noticeably quiet; she was thinking about how her own child had started to develop emotional problems during her own hospital admission for a medical condition.

This led on to a discussion about Diane's own theories about why Patrick behaved as he did. Initially she said she hadn't a clue and she added that she was here for the doctors to tell her why he was 'mental' and that she wouldn't have come to the unit if she hadn't been told she had to by her 'awful' social worker. However, the group facilitators gently encouraged her to think whether any of the earlier questions might give her some clues about her son's emotional state. She said she had wondered whether he had ADHD (attention deficit hyperactivity disorder) and that she had been disappointed when the paediatrician said he did not. She also wondered if he was attention-seeking. She'd rejected the latter idea, as she knew she gave him more attention than any of her other children. This led to a group discussion about whether children stopped seeking attention when they were given it and whether it made a difference if the attention they received was positive or negative.

The facilitator had wondered whether to ask Diane about a possible link between Patrick's behaviour and his experience of sexual abuse but she decided not to as Diane was so tense and anxious. However, David's mum had obviously had the same thought and felt confident enough to ask. Diane thought about this for a while and eventually said that it might be an important factor – but clearly this was a difficult idea for her to think about. Indeed this issue had come up in a recent family therapy session and she had dismissed the idea out of hand.

The group listened carefully to Diane as she talked about trying different ways to control Patrick. She said she had smacked him when he was younger but since the social care department had become involved she had been told not to do this. She felt that Patrick had picked up on this and had in fact threatened to tell the social worker if she so much as raised her hand to him.

She'd also tried some star charts, as suggested – but they'd only worked for a week – and Patrick had torn them up and told her he 'didn't care if he never got any stars'.

The session was drawing to a close – usually the facilitators would encourage the parent to identify a strategy to try during the week but in Diane's case she seemed so fragile that they felt she might be too overwhelmed to try any new strategies that week. However, Diane was able to talk more about the circumstances around the potential abuse during the week, and she came more confidently to the following week's session.

Trips out

At the end of each week there is a group for all the families that involves a trip off the unit site; the activity could be going swimming, or bowling, or to a local wildlife centre. Sometimes it might involve a trip to a local supermarket to buy the ingredients for a cooking session. This group gives staff and families a chance to be outside the contained, controlled environment of the unit. The group is eagerly anticipated by the children, but often parents feel quite anxious about managing their children in a public space. Often prior to admission parents have stopped taking their children to these places because of difficult and embarrassing experiences. Again parents find tackling this challenge as a group much more approachable than if they were trying it on their own.

The focus of this session is to encourage positive family interactions and to increase each family's confidence that they can manage everyday activities. The staff have to make sure that children will be safe during these trips, so children will be aware that their behaviour on the unit during the week will help the staff to be confident that they can be safe during this trip. During the last week of their stay children are allowed to choose the activity for this group. This is part of the leaving ritual. Often children have very strong memories of the fun of these trips out.

Summary

This chapter has focused on the practice of multi-family work in the setting of a children's inpatient unit. Whilst this setting is not a common one, the majority of the principles and ideas discussed would have applicability in a wider range of settings, where more than one family (or a family member) come together in a group setting. The clinical experience of the unit reflects the literature about this therapeutic approach and confirms that it is a particularly beneficial approach for families with children who have complex needs.

Chapter 6

Accessing Learning

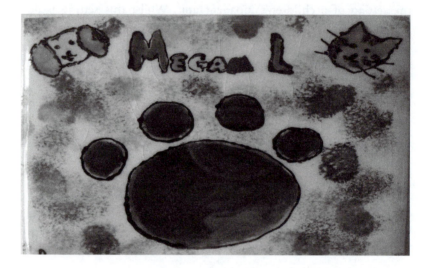

*The animals Megan drew reminded her of the
stickers that she received in school*

Introduction

As one might expect, children with mental health problems usually
experience difficulties in all settings. However, schooling presents
particular challenges and may be, for some, where their difficulties
are most evident. Formal schooling in the UK starts at five years of
age and over the last decade schooling has become dominated by a
National Curriculum which focuses on achieving set targets. Children
are formally tested from a very young age and there has been a shift
in primary teaching away from child-centred learning to a more
standardised approach.

Children with emotional and/or behavioural problems and children
with developmental disorders often need higher levels of nurture and
support than their peers and may also need a differentiated curriculum.
This puts a great demand on the host school to meet their individual

needs. The increasing formalisation of schooling has run alongside a trend to reduce places in special schools and an expectation that mainstream schools will accommodate children with a very wide range of sensory, learning and emotional difficulties who in earlier decades would have been schooled in specialist centres.

Almost invariably the children who need specialist intensive mental health treatment will have had considerable difficulties in their school placements. In the UK there was a dramatic increase in the rates of exclusions for primary-aged children in the late 1990s (Parsons 1998), and considerable efforts are now being made to reverse this trend.

Often children accessing inpatient care arrive with a very negative and anxious experience of being in a classroom. And yet we know that academic achievements and ongoing engagement in training are key factors in developing resilience and emotional wellbeing for children and young people, particularly those with risk factors such as parents with mental illness or substance misuse problems (Daniel, Wassell and Gilligan 1999). For many parents, their child's failure in the education system will be one of their main concerns, and finding the optimal school placement or additional support will be a major aim.

So the educational programme at the Croft is not just a legal requirement but a key element of the therapeutic plan to re-engage the children in ordinary daily life and to give them opportunities to succeed. This chapter describes the school unit within the Croft and how reluctant, anxious learners are supported to re-engage with the educational process.

All children of school age who are admitted to the Croft attend the unit school in the mornings. School at the Croft operates at several levels. Many children who come to the Croft have been excluded from mainstream (and sometimes even special) schools due to their inability to conform to behavioural and social expectations. Others may have been refusing to attend school after traumatic experiences at school or because of difficulties separating from their parents. Frequently children have not attended school for extended periods of time – a year or sometimes even longer – and have often become more and more socially isolated whilst receiving part-time teaching at home. Some younger children are just managing to maintain mainstream placements but increasingly struggling as the cognitive demands of the curriculum become more complex, requiring self-direction and organisation. Others struggle with friendships which require more social competence than they may have. There is also a small group of children (particularly those suffering from eating disorders) who may appear to be very successful at school, being motivated and achieving highly, but in other ways often find maintaining their own high standards and need for perfection increasingly stressful.

Providing continuity

A primary role of the teacher in child and family psychiatric settings is to provide continuity of education for all the children who are admitted, but the classroom setting also provides a valuable part of the assessment process. How children function in a small educational group setting academically, socially, behaviourally and emotionally, are all questions that can be considered. Some children who come to the Croft (particularly those diagnosed with attention deficit hyperactivity disorder, ADHD) will be on medication during their admission, and the classroom setting is an ideal place to observe the effect on attention and impulsivity of changing the dosages of a medication or trying a different type of medication. The ability to share and work co-operatively within a group is also demonstrated within this setting.

Many children are extremely negative about schools, having previously failed in at least one school or having had a long and difficult history of short-term exclusions. Most children have not managed to establish secure friendship groups in their home schools and feel socially isolated within the classroom and playground. Children on the autistic spectrum may have found school to be an extremely challenging environment, struggling with not being able to follow their own agenda, doing things in their way that makes sense to them and having been regarded as 'odd' by their peers.

The resulting low self-esteem, anxiety and social isolation mean that for many children school has become an extremely difficult and unhappy place. Many have developed their own coping strategies such as avoidance of failure by difficult behaviour or using provocative clowning behaviour, to interact with peers and to draw attention to themselves.

The National Curriculum and achievement levels

The school at the Croft is funded and managed by the local education department. Together with the school provision at the neighbouring adolescent unit (The Darwin Centre), eating disorders unit (The Phoenix Centre) and Addenbrooke's Hospital, it forms the Medical Pupil Referral Unit (PRU), called the Pilgrim PRU. The PRU is regularly inspected by Ofsted (Office for Standards in Education) and at the last inspection (2009) it was judged to be outstanding in its provision. The National Curriculum forms the core of the curriculum at the Croft and children are assessed against curriculum levels on admission and on discharge to measure progress using an online assessment package called 'Goal' (see www.goalonline.co.uk). This can provide an instant picture of the child's current level of achievement and is particularly useful for those who have been outside of the school system for lengthy periods of time. For younger children or those working below National Curriculum levels, the online Smart Cat (published by Screen Learning; see www.screenlearning.com) assessment provides a useful picture of their strengths and weaknesses and is seen by most children as an enjoyable computer game. These are very useful tools in a classroom where the average length of stay is six weeks and enable the teacher to immediately identify areas of weakness for each individual child and to maximise their learning within such a short timeframe.

Links with the children's existing schools

An additional role for the teacher is to liaise with the child's current school (if he has one). The child's own teacher's perspective always provides additional insights into his difficulties. The unit teacher can also act in a consultative manner to the child's school at the end of the admission, using observations and insights gained during the admission to support his re-integration back into his local school. In some cases the unit teaching staff play a key role in helping children re-integrate into their original school or into a new school placement. This may mean that one of the teaching assistants or a member of the nursing team accompanies a child for a few sessions as he returns to a mainstream environment – thus ensuring that information about the child and his care is transferred to the school. The presence of a staff member from the unit can also ease the anxiety of the child, his family and the school.

Sometimes a child may have been functioning very well in his own school prior to admission, as the school may have been a haven for the child from family conflict or other difficulties. In this case it may be appropriate for the child to continue to attend his own school for one day a week during his admission, in order to maintain the existing positive relationships.

The physical environment

The Croft school is integrated with the rest of the unit, and it is situated within the same building. However, when children enter the classroom doors at the beginning of the day it is important that they see it as a separate environment with the expectations and norms of a school. This can be difficult for some children with separation difficulties as they are aware that their parents are just on the other side of the school door. Conversely some children find this immensely reassuring, and the fact that they know that mum will be available for a quick hug at playtime is instrumental in helping them to settle into the classroom.

The school consists of two well-resourced classrooms, a school office, access to the adjacent art room and a useful cooling down area known as 'the lobby'. One classroom is used for the main teaching parts of the morning and the second contains computers and a wide variety of activities such as construction toys, sand and water play, a role-play area, puzzles, games and books. These are used as part of a reward system that includes earning a short free choice when a piece of work has been completed to the satisfaction of teaching staff, and form a vital part of motivating children to work in the classroom.

There are three adults working within the classroom: one teacher and two teaching assistants. This is a well-established team who have developed a structure and ways of working together within the classroom over the last 18 years.

A varied curriculum

As the unit admits children aged across the primary age range and beyond, some children being 13 years old and occasionally even older, the school has to manage a wide range of ages. All the children are taught within the same classroom and it is not unusual to have a five-year-old and a 13-year-old within the same group. Whilst this sounds like a very wide age gap, frequently the older children are still working within the primary school curriculum levels and are socially and emotionally immature. The aim will often be to teach the same curriculum topic in literacy and science, for example covering a topic like measurement in different ways in different subjects. In addition, the age and ability range necessitates a huge amount of differentiation within the classroom, with, for example, one child struggling to form one or two words to describe a picture illustrating the same subject about which another child is writing several pages and another using a laptop computer to compose a short passage.

Literacy is often a particular challenge for many of the children, and particularly for the boys. Many have identified, specific literacy difficulties and they have often well-established oppositional behaviour patterns which emerge when they are asked to write. The aim is always to provide children with a way to gradually achieve some amount of success and enjoyment with writing, valuing and praising all efforts. Much of this is done, as with all work, through display. A crumpled torn-up scruffy piece of paper can be smoothed, sellotaped, mounted beautifully and transformed into a success. An illegible passage of writing can be word-processed and illustrated by the child, furthering ICT skills at the same time as producing a legible piece of work.

Story time

Many children have no tradition of story reading at home and one of the parts of the school morning enjoyed by almost all the children is listening to a story. This is a wonderful time, taking place after mid-morning break, when the children often return unsettled from the excitement and social difficulties of the playground. As the teacher starts to read, the children quickly relax and forget their conflicts as they become involved in the world of the book. Amazingly even the most hyperactive and disruptive children are often able to sit calmly to listen to a 20-minute story. Those who find it hard not to fidget and fiddle whilst listening are offered the option of drawing whilst they listen and interesting pictures, often following the theme of the story, materialise during this time. It is extremely gratifying that many children go on to ask their parents to buy them books that have been read in the classroom and this demonstrates to the parents that their children can get pleasure from being read to rather than just watching cartoons or DVDs.

Rewarding achievements and building up self-esteem

There is a comprehensive reward system within the classroom that runs throughout each session. Every week, each child has a cardboard cut-out shape such as a dog or an aeroplane, often chosen by the children, on a chart on the wall. The stickers that they earn for getting to the classroom on time, doing what the grown-ups say and getting on with their work are collected throughout the week. There is also a separate sticker reward for good language, that is, not using rude words or swear words or saying unkind things, something many of the children struggle with. The adults award the stickers at the end of each session and the ritual of going to the teacher's desk to receive stickers is adhered to strictly. The children watch each other as they take it in turns to go up to the teacher, and they hear the positive comments made to each child in turn. The children then wear the stickers on their clothing throughout the rest of the day to show their parents and the staff how well they are doing in class. A sufficiency of stickers at the end of the week (and there is always the possibility of regaining lost ground by earning a bonus for trying especially hard) earns a small reward such as a pencil sharpener, pen, badge, and so on. This system of rewards is highly (and often surprisingly) motivating, and often the reminder of a sticker is enough to produce compliance.

Running alongside the sticker reward system is the motivation of earning a free choice – the chance to choose an activity when a piece of work has been completed satisfactorily. This is enormously motivating and works on several different levels. Many of the children are overactive and struggle to sit still, or may still be at a developmental stage where, in a reception classroom, they would be in a play-based environment. Being able to get up, move around and choose an appealing activity allows these children self-directed time before returning to an adult-directed activity. Free choice time is differentiated and adjusted according to the age and need of each individual child, recognising that a five-year-old or overactive child needs a much more frequent break than a 12-year-old.

Free choice time also offers an opportunity to observe how each child functions socially: do they choose solo activities or do they repetitively choose (as many autistic children do) the same activity? Do they play imaginatively in the role-play area? Do they play with other children or only relate to adults? What happens to the family figures in the dolls' house? How do they use the sand play trays? All these observations contribute to the team task of building a picture of the children's patterns of behaviour.

Free time is also a chance to sit and chat to an adult about their fears and worries whilst playing with LEGO or other construction toys. Often the children reveal their low self-esteem as they talk about problems in their local schools, and many talk about having been bullied. Some describe their awareness of being unable to perform like their peers and their resulting social exclusion.

Challenging behaviours

Challenging behaviour is extremely common amongst the children who come to the Croft. Physical aggression such as kicking, hitting, biting, spitting and throwing equipment and verbal aggression such as shouting and swearing are often displayed within the classroom. Some children have previously found that antisocial behaviour leads to a positive outcome, for example, an adult no longer asking them to complete their work or being sent home from the school environment – the very place that they hate.

Children who come to the unit are often surprised to discover that difficult behaviour does not automatically lead to them being excluded from the classroom. Whilst the classroom does have an emergency buzzer system to summon help if a child's behaviour becomes too risky to manage, huge efforts are made to keep children in the classroom at all times and to contain their behaviour. Many children have learning difficulties and are working well below their chronological ages. Many have poor fine motor skills and find recording their work laborious and difficult and therefore seek ways to avoid it. Motivating children to put pencil to paper is often a challenging and time-consuming task but one that is very rewarding, both for the child and adult, when they realise little by little that they are making progress. All work is carefully preserved to enable children to see their own progress.

Many children with emotional and attachment problems are very needy of adult attention, therefore attention-seeking behaviour is also extremely common in the classroom. This may be manifested in negative behaviours such as calling out, banging on the tables, falling off chairs, rolling on the floor, and so on. Some children need the reassurance of an adult close by and just sitting beside their table can often give the security and reassurance needed to enable them to settle to work. Children with insecure attachments often crave physical closeness and will either seek this by constantly asking for help that they do not actually need or by behaving in a way that requires an adult to sit with them. Many children seeking physical contact want to cuddle up to staff which can be a difficult issue in a classroom context. Conversely children on the autistic spectrum often find physical closeness very uncomfortable which makes tasks such as hearing these children read quite a challenge. Teaching staff have to be aware of the needs of each individual child and to be able to adopt the optimal level of physical closeness and nurturing for each child whilst encouraging their own emotional self-management skills to develop.

Friendships and group dynamics

Establishing friendships and managing social interactions are huge issues for the children. Many children on leaving the unit will say that one of the best things about their stay has been having a friend for the first time. This reflects the importance of a friendship group for a child's happiness and mental wellbeing. However, working co-operatively within a group, taking turns and sharing equipment are challenges for many of the children. Although the classroom is arranged so that all the children have an identified, individual work space, whenever possible the children also work together as a group at times sharing space, equipment and ideas. The amount of group work that the children can manage is dependent on a number of factors, for example, their ages, social skills and level of emotional containment.

Teaching staff are frequently amazed at how well the children adapt to working around a peer's disruptive behaviour, stepping over upturned furniture and equipment or ignoring wailing and banging as if they were part of ordinary everyday life (as indeed they often are at the Croft). Children will sometimes voice their sympathy for their peers when they are having difficulties and will sometimes also state that it is reassuring for them to know that others have difficult times as well as themselves.

As new children arrive almost weekly, it is a regular challenge for the children and staff to integrate them into the school group. Children who have worked together for a number of weeks learn to accommodate each other's difficulties, whether they consist of anxiety, frequent twitches or explosive behaviours. However, each new arrival can cause anxiety and disruption to the group dynamics.

As in all group environments, children quickly establish roles within the group. New children are quickly quizzed as to when their birthdays are, the oldest child being anxious to preserve his superiority within the group. Younger children often find they enjoy the role of being looked after by an older child who feels less threatened playing with younger children than with his same age peers.

A further aspect of the group dynamic is that although the majority of the children are resident, a small number attend daily. These children may have been resident during the early part of their admission or may be fairly local children who can attend as day-patients. The residential children socialise together in the evening and day children may feel excluded from this group. Children who have been resident but subsequently become day-patients often miss the residential setting with all the opportunities this offers for activities with staff and other children to play with, and they may resent the fact that other children have taken their place and are sleeping in 'their' bedroom.

A morning in school

A morning in school is never dull and it presents a constantly changing challenge to the teaching staff. There is a consistent need to be flexible and to react quickly to the emotional state of the children, creating an environment that not only moves children forward in their learning, but enables children to improve their self-esteem, to foster positive relationships with teachers and teaching assistants and to begin to find some enjoyment in being in a classroom. This variety and constant need to adapt to different needs and unexpected challenges makes the teaching job stimulating and highly satisfying.

Many children find moving from one part of the programme to another (what staff refer to as transitions) particularly difficult. Moving from the short play at the beginning of the day and arriving outside the classroom door in an orderly line is something that sounds simple but can be fraught with opportunities for conflict.

> At 9.30, Wendy, the teacher, has already attended the morning handover meeting with the Croft team, been part of the morning meeting with the children and updated the two teaching assistants Anne and Susan P, explaining what to expect from the children on that day. Wendy, Anne and Susan are ready for the school morning to begin. As happens frequently the children lining up outside the door are noisy and Anne waits for them to settle down before opening the door. She notices that Nick is wearing his baseball hat and leaning against the wall scowling rather than standing in line. Arthur is agitated and unsettled by the presence of this new peer. Patrick has run back to the residential area to find his mother, closely followed by a member of the nursing team. David stands with Philippa, who is carefully holding a brand new pencil case.
>
> Patrick is retrieved and the line settles enough for Anne to open the door and be first to greet the children. She notices Nick's baseball cap which he has refused to hand over to nursing staff. Wendy asks him to remove his hat; initially he refuses and swears before giving in and throwing the hat out of the door. He is hyper-vigilant and anxious, pacing around the room and kicking over his chair. Arthur continues to grumble about Nick, saying that he is making his head ache. Philippa is clearly anxious that staff should notice her lovely new pencil case, complete with themed pens and pencils, and she places it ostentatiously on the edge of her table. David and Patrick settle down although Patrick rocks backwards and forwards on his chair watching Nick with some admiration. Gradually order is restored. Nick is reminded about the boundaries

in the classroom and that the adults know that new situations are difficult and he is asked if there is anything that will help him settle. Although he continues to swear he picks his chair up and sits down.

Arthur is very unsettled by Nick's behaviour and Susan asks him if he is worried about Nick. Arthur cannot acknowledge that the arrival of a new peer is difficult for him and just says he feels tired. Nevertheless, he is calmed by reminders of how well he has been doing in class and that he will be able to use his favourite computer program for a free choice if he gets on with the work that he has been given. Computer programs are the thing that Arthur likes best and therefore help to motivate him to work hard. Other children may have other favourite activities, such as playing in the sand, for example.

Philippa's pencil case is duly noted and admired.

The children are asked individually to fetch their work trays and tuck their chairs in as they leave their table, establishing the expectation that things should be done in a calm and orderly manner. This passes without incident apart from Nick, crashing his tray down with a huge bang, making Philippa and David jump.

The children are at last ready to start work: they are currently working on traditional stories. The literacy lesson is looking at the idea of character in these stories. A discussion starts about the characters that the children remember from fairy stories. Arthur and Patrick both enthusiastically launch into a description of various characters they know from the Shrek DVD – they talk over each other and cannot listen to one another and boundaries have to be set. Patrick sulks and Arthur grins. Philippa reels off a long and accurate list of appropriate characters. David adds a few token comments and Nick refuses to co-operate before grudgingly adding that he used to watch Snow White with his gran.

Having managed to compile quite a comprehensive list on the board, the children watch a PowerPoint presentation on the whiteboard. This goes well as most of the children who come to the Croft respond well to information presented visually, and attractive presentations using different media, including film clips, hold their interest. Arthur gets up and starts dancing to the music, Nick jeers at him, he responds to Susan's request to sit down and she moves to sit near him to help him focus. As the whiteboard presentation finishes Wendy outlines the next part of the task to the children. As usual they struggle to listen and even after repeating the simple instructions twice, Arthur and Patrick both ask what they have to do. After many repeated questions and rummaging around for books, pencils, and so on, everyone has the right equipment and begins to create their own character for a fairy story.

Nick states that he is going to draw a character from Grand Theft Auto. When told this won't be acceptable he swears at Anne and tears up his piece of paper, scowling and resentful. Anne fetches him a fresh piece of paper, sits down besides him and engages him in chatting about his favourite football team (as evidenced by the sweat bands she has noticed he is wearing), before swiftly moving on to helping him to think about what sort of character he might attempt. He grudgingly agrees to create a monster and quickly reveals that he is actually quite a talented artist. The adults all quietly praise his picture and he cannot help grinning.

The next 20 minutes pass reasonably calmly with the usual provision of plenty of support and positive encouragement to keep everyone on task and moving forward. The children gradually finish the task to the best of their ability. Patrick finishes first and is given much praise for his efforts and the reward of a free choice. He chooses to make a LEGO model and moves to sit in the adjacent room where he is quickly joined by Nick. Anne goes to sit with them to help them manage being close to one another and sharing the same box of equipment. Nick immediately begins boasting about his skill at making LEGO models and how much LEGO he has at home. Anne quickly moves the conversation on before an argument develops and she finds herself receiving a long description of Nick's favourite motorbike.

Susan P continues to support Arthur who has chosen to draw and write about a dragon. He is very involved in a detailed drawing, carefully outlining every scale on the body and rapidly running out of time to complete the writing part of the task. When Susan attempts to suggest he should move on to the writing he is rude and resistant, insisting he has to finish the drawing first. They reach a compromise when Susan P reminds him of the sticker she wants him to earn and reassures him that there'll be time to finish his drawing whilst listening to the story after breaktime. He begins his writing with Susan's help.

Playtime is approaching and those children who are having a free choice are reminded that they have two minutes left before they need to clear up. Those children who are still working are asked to find a suitable stopping place. Philippa replaces her beautiful pens and pencils neatly in her pencil case and sits quietly whilst the rest of the group gradually shuffle papers, pencils and equipment into work trays. After several reminders the children achieve reasonable order and eventually they are all waiting quietly to be chosen to come up for their sticker. Noticing that Arthur is making a big effort to be still, Wendy calls him up first. As he leaves his place he glances at Nick to make sure that he has noticed that he is first. Arthur's morning is discussed with him and he appears unusually pleased with the praise he receives, making good eye contact and smiling. The rest of the group follow one by one to get their feedback before lining up for play. As they line up there is the usual shuffling and jostling until they are reminded that they need to be in a straight quiet line before they can go to play. The door is opened; the children rush out to the waiting nurses who escort them to the playground, and Wendy, Anne and Susan go for a well-earned cup of coffee...

Summary

This chapter set out to describe the issues around helping complex children access learning and how the observations and activities in school contribute to the overall assessment and therapeutic plan. The schoolroom plays a vital part in the rehabilitation of children who are fearful and avoidant, and the structure, containment and nurturing discussed in the previous chapters are all illustrated by the approach used by the experienced and sensitive teaching staff.

Atypical features of the Croft classroom include the close proximity of parents, and the diverse nature of the children in terms of their developmental ages, their difficulties and the rapidly changing composition of the group. These aspects, as indicated, present both opportunities and challenges.

Although there are unusual aspects to the teaching setting of the Croft, many of the techniques used will be familiar to experienced special needs teachers. Increasingly mainstream teachers are being asked to accommodate children with complex mental health needs in a large classroom, so it is to be hoped that the ideas presented in this chapter will be thought-provoking and useful.

Chapter 7

Fostering the Child's Social World

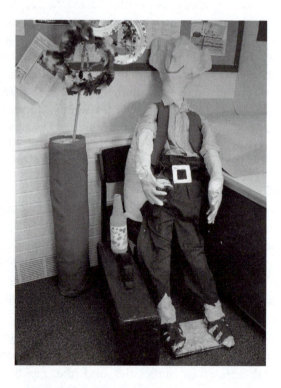

The BFG created in the art group

Introduction

Humans are social creatures and social connectedness is increasingly recognised as a vital component of good mental health. Positive family and peer relationships form resilience factors for children (and adults) who are exposed to traumatic events. In contrast, most of the children who are admitted to mental health units have significant problems with interpersonal relationships. Typically the children find it difficult to communicate emotionally, they try to control relationships and they find sharing and compromise a huge challenge. They often have complicated and difficult relationships within their families and usually have few or no friends.

Sometimes these social interaction difficulties are inherent characteristics of the child, as in the case of children with an autistic spectrum disorder, and sometimes they arise as a consequence of adverse environmental circumstances. In the case of children with severe and complex needs, their lack of social competence is often a consequence of the interaction of both genetic and social disadvantage.

One of the fundamental roles of an intensive mental health assessment is to describe the children's strengths and difficulties in detail. Some children, for example those with milder forms of autism, may not show their difficulties in outpatient-based, one-to-one situations, as they may be very able to communicate with supportive adults. But the same children may have very significant social problems when they are with their peers. For these children, it is essential to work with them in group situations, in order to see the range of their abilities and to foster their social competence (Richer and Coates 2001).

Children who have experienced abusive relationships may well relate to others in inappropriate ways, whilst others may feel embarrassed in front of their peers because they have tics or poor language skills. Some children take on the role of class clown or use babyish behaviour in order to establish a relationship with their peers. These behaviours, designed to mask the primary problem, may become a 'secondary handicap', as described by Valerie Sinason (1992), creating even greater hurdles for the children as they attempt to establish positive age-appropriate friendships.

Many of the children seen in child and family psychiatric units will have experienced teasing and bullying and some will have been bullies themselves. Most of the children talk of feeling isolated and alone and of how they long for friends (Lines 2007). Due to the high levels of specialist adult support and focus on group activities, inpatient psychiatric units have a privileged opportunity to help children relate to their peers in positive ways, and to help them to regain confidence in their abilities to socialise and interact with others. Nevertheless, this can be a hugely challenging task as most of the children within the group have similar problems and group situations can very easily spiral out of control. Staff often have to think creatively to provide group experiences that will suit a wide range of children of varying ages with different needs and abilities. The nature of inpatient units is that there are children arriving and leaving almost every week, so the composition of the group will vary from week to week. This creates an additional challenge as often staff will prepare material for a group only to find that the children's needs have changed, the atmosphere in the group is different to the previous week and what might have been appropriate the week before is no longer suitable. Staff often have to think on their feet, reacting in the moment to changing needs.

Due to the multi-family group setting, children will be in the unusual situation of living with their peer group and members of their family simultaneously. This in itself is a very socially stimulating environment but it could be confusing for some children who might want to keep school or daytime relationships with their peers separate from family relationships. If children have been displaying very different behaviours in and outside their home, this may help them to change their usual patterns of behaviour and become more integrated in their relatedness. Another issue that some children will address during group therapeutic activities with their peers is that of control. They are asked to accept the adults' authority and to share attention with their peers.

This chapter describes some of the groups and social situations provided for the children at the Croft. The group programme consists of a variety of therapeutic approaches, some creative, some cognitive and some physical in their focus. They are designed to tap into different domains, and comparing how a child interacts in a music therapy setting to her functioning in a social skills group can be very informative and show different patterns of strengths and difficulties. Children love to interact with their friends in fun activities and the groups can help to rebuild their confidence in their ability to cope in social situations and to make friends. For children who have been out of school for months or years, just being able to cope with a full day of social contact will be a major achievement and may be the first step back into education.

Some groups have been running for a long time and form the stable skeleton of the group programme; others may be varied or created to meet the varying needs of the children. As described in Chapter 3, the group programme works alongside the school sessions to provide a predictable daily structure for the children. There is routine and repetition within the group sessions, such as starting each group with a reminder of 'the rules'; again this re-emphasises the structure, helping children to orientate to the groups quickly and assimilate the adult's expectations of them within the group.

Social skills group

Since many children who are admitted to psychiatric services struggle in their relationships with their peers, a social skills group that directly addresses these difficulties seems an important element of treatment. The social skills group currently run at the Croft is based on a positive approach where the focus is on the children's strengths rather than on their difficulties (Drost 2006).

The topics in this group are challenging: bullying, anger, friendship and loneliness. However, these often emotive subjects are presented in an approachable and non-confrontational way. The group is very structured and mixes use of worksheets with games and relaxation. The group uses cognitive behavioural techniques to help children identify feelings, both their own and those of other people.

Parents sometimes observe the sessions from behind a one-way screen accompanied by a member of staff, and this is made clear to the children. This is part of the multi-family approach (see Chapter 5). This provides a very useful opportunity for parents as they will rarely have seen their child working with other children in a group focused on social and emotional communication. Some will be surprised at how insightful their child can be, and it can be an opportunity for staff to focus on positive aspects of children's progress.

> Colleen, Andrew, Mark and Phil (nurses) plan the social skills group. They decide to focus on 'what makes us angry', remembering that in the previous week Nick had been unable to think about his own anger and Philippa had denied that she ever experienced anger. They allocate Mark to support Nick and explain to Nick before the group that Mark will be helping him.
>
> Colleen, Andrew and Mark sit on the floor waiting for the children to be brought to the group therapy room. Phil takes the

parents into the observation booth. Nick, Patrick, Philippa and David rush in excitedly as they have just finished a game of tag during the break. Philippa immediately settles down but the boys take a little while to settle. Once everyone is quiet Andrew reminds the children that the parents are behind the screen with Phil. Patrick immediately gets up and peers through the one-way screen attempting to see his mother. Nick runs up and joins him, they both make silly gestures and shout for a minute or so. Staff ignore their behaviour and talk quietly to Philippa and David, praising their attention. Eventually Patrick and Nick tire of the one-way screen and come to sit down.

Colleen asks the children in turn to tell her one of the rules of the group – Philippa is asked to write them on the whiteboard so that everyone can see them throughout the group. She writes:

1. Hands and feet to yourself

2. No interrupting

3. Listen to each other

4. Be proud of what you do

5. Have fun

Colleen reminds the children about what they did in the previous week's group. She reminds them of what they had said about anger and she remembers that Patrick told the group that he shouts when he's angry, and that the children (except for Philippa) had all agreed that they also shout when they're angry.

At this point Arthur comes in looking sad. He apologises for being late. Colleen welcomes him to the group and explains what they have done so far. Philippa says she never feels angry but sometimes feels sad. Andrew asks the children whether they sometimes feel angry and sad at the same time.

Mark introduces the funny walks game. He suggests they all try walking around the room in a sad way, then in an angry way. Nick then suggests they walk around as though they were drunk. His walk is realistic and makes everyone laugh.

Colleen then suggests that they might want to think about different levels of anger and introduces a worksheet where children are encouraged to draw a thermometer with numbers. The children are asked to write on the thermometer things that make them angry, thinking about things that make them a little irritable to things that make them furious. Mark works with Nick who starts off by writing at the bottom of the thermometer about his little brother who takes his favourite toy cars and scratches them. Further up the thermometer he writes 'my headteacher always thinks it is my fault'. Nick hesitates when Mark asks him what he is going to put at the top of his thermometer – he looks sad and starts chewing the pencil. Eventually he writes 'my Mum' but almost as soon as he has written the words he scribbles them out.

Philippa is working with Colleen – at first she just sits doing nothing and says she cannot think of anything to write. Colleen tries to help her out by talking about everyday things that make her angry, hoping to show Philippa that being angry is an ordinary emotion. Philippa still cannot name anything at home that makes her angry but she manages to acknowledge that Patrick made her 'a bit cross' earlier on in the day because he said her hair was messy. She then says that the staff made her feel 'a bit cross' when she first came to the unit by telling her she had to finish her meals and that she had felt very scared too. Colleen asked her whether she still feels angry and scared about eating – Philippa thinks hard about this and then says she doesn't often feel angry any more but she still feels scared that the staff are trying to make her fat. Colleen praises Philippa for being brave and talking about her feelings, and acknowledges how difficult her feelings must be to cope with. Colleen and Philippa talk a little about the strategies that Philippa has been working on with the psychologist to cope with her fear of becoming fat.

At the end of the group Mark encourages the children to lie on the floor and relax. He tells them a story where someone is angry and worried and then a story where someone is happy and relaxed. As the children listen to the stories he asks them to notice how their bodies feel, how fast they are breathing and how tense their muscles are.

When Colleen, Andrew, Mark and Phil meet later in the day, they discuss how pleased they are that the children all managed to remain in the room for 45 minutes. They note in particular that Nick was starting to acknowledge some of his feelings and that Philippa seemed much more open about her fears.

Art group

The art group takes place early on in the week. Most children feel comfortable in an art activity because it will be a very familiar format to art activities they have done in their own schools. Because it is a creative group it has a lower verbal demand than other groups and can be operated on several levels, depending on the children's needs. Some children particularly like art and feel confident in this area. Others will gain a sense of achievement from being helped to produce something tangible that they feel good about and that they can see being valued by adults and peers. Other children will gain pleasure and satisfaction from using art materials in very basic tactile ways, for example, finger painting and clay work. For many children, particularly those on the autistic spectrum, using messy materials such as paint and glue poses a particular difficulty and the art group can provide a gentle introduction where they can begin to overcome these difficulties (Buchalter 2009).

Children may also recreate some of their experiences through the art activity. In family portraits it can be revealing to see which members of the family are included in the picture. Other children may have strong themes to their artwork, such as scenes of aggression or catastrophe.

At the Croft, the art group is run by the unit teacher (Wendy), a teaching assistant (Anne) and a nurse (Alan). This group provides a cross-over into school as it is run jointly by teaching and nursing staff. The artwork is often planned to fit in with the school curriculum. Thus the aims of the art group are both therapeutic and educational. The art group is the first group of the week and provides a gentle and non-threatening start to the group programme.

> In school the children have been reading the BFG by Roald Dahl (Dahl 1982). Over several weeks in art group, the children have created a large papier-mâché model of the giant. This week the children will be painting the model. Nick enters the room scowling. He refuses to put on an apron, saying it is 'babyish'. Wendy suggests that he wear one of the grown-up aprons but he still refuses. Anne tries to distract him by asking him to help Arthur to get his apron on. She then reminds him that without an apron nobody can take part. He sits in a corner and sulks, kicking a chair.

Philippa, on the other hand, is really enjoying herself. She spontaneously helps Arthur who is tentative about holding the paintbrush because he hates getting any paint on his hands. When it comes to doing her own painting she focuses on one of the BFG's eyes, meticulously painting each detail. Wendy praises her but also suggests she might move on to using a bigger brush to paint his arms. Philippa needs help to be bold and experiment and not get stuck on intricate details.

Alan is working with Patrick and trying to stop him from being distracted by Nick's grumpy behaviour. He is also encouraging Patrick to put the paint on the BFG rather than all over his own arms and face. At this point Anne takes Nick aside to a separate table, hands him his apron, and suggests that he put it on, so that he can help paint the BFG's suitcase which is a special project which requires a slightly older and more responsible child. Nick accepts this task and starts painting.

The BFG project continued over several weeks. At the end the children make invitations for staff and their families to come to a 'grand unveiling' of the BFG. All the children take part in the preparations for the party and they serve home-made 'frobscottle' and 'snozzcumbers' to the adults with great aplomb. On several occasions Nick points out the BFG's suitcase to his mum and to staff and he proudly tells them that he painted it on his own.

Music therapy group

The music therapist, Amelia, has worked at the Croft for over 20 years. The music therapy group is for all the children on the unit and has been a weekly event since the establishment of music therapy on the unit. The children are generally motivated to play the instruments and usually enjoy the session. In the group all the children and the adults can make music together through free improvisation, often facilitated by Amelia at the piano. This means that children of different ages with different levels of abilities as well as the adults can play together as equals. Children who struggle with words can interact with one another non-verbally.

Music making can give children an opportunity to be 'little' or playful, which they may struggle to do in other groups without being embarrassed. The music group is often a stimulating and exciting environment where children will behave differently from other settings and show sides of themselves they do not show elsewhere. However, because of the heightened levels of arousal in this group, some children will struggle to behave in appropriate ways, and managing the group is not always easy.

Further information about music therapy at the Croft is available. This group has already been described in detail with reference to case studies of specific children taking part in the group (Oldfield 2006). The specific role that the music therapy group plays in the diagnosis of the children's strengths and difficulties has also been explored previously (Carter and Oldfield 2002).

> As Amelia heaves the drum kit and some of the larger instruments out of the music room to make room for eight small chairs arranged in a circle, events from the previous week's music group flash through her brain. Arthur came in late and then refused to sit in the chair that was suggested for him, saying he wanted to be next to the cupboard. When the adults insisted he should sit on his allocated chair, he kicked over the chair and became quite aggressive, which led to him being asked to leave the room. Later he returned and was able to enjoy some of the group playing. Amelia wonders whether he had felt a little confined and claustrophobic in the position that had been chosen for him...she decides to try positioning him in the seat he wanted the previous week. She also remembers that it was difficult not to overlook Philippa, as she was so compliant and quiet. Amelia makes a mental note to see what she is doing and perhaps even to ask her to lead an activity.
>
> Susan, a member of the nursing team, arrives to help Amelia prepare for the group. She tells Amelia that Nick and Patrick have had to be separated in the playground outside earlier that day. Patrick desperately wants Nick to be his friend but Nick easily loses patience with Patrick and often teases him, which frequently results in Patrick becoming aggressive. They also both wonder whether Patrick is finding this week particularly difficult because he knows it is his last week on the unit and is sad about leaving. They decide to seat them on either side of Susan, who reminds Amelia that staff have noticed David muttering to himself and that they should look out for any verbal or facial tics. This will help the medical team

to decide whether or not he should be diagnosed with Tourette's syndrome.

As the children spill into the room, they are quickly encouraged to sit in the places that Susan and Amelia feel will work best for them all. Arthur seems relieved to have been allocated the seat he coveted the previous week. Amelia welcomes the children and reminds them that it is a special group because it is Patrick's last week. He looks cross and says 'Hurrah! Can't wait to go…' but this is not very convincing.

Amelia starts the 'hello' activity where the children copy her beats on the Bodhran drum and she tries to catch them out by stopping in unexpected places. The drum is then passed on to a child who then becomes the leader and tries to catch others out. It is the beginning of the session and the children generally enjoy this activity where there is an element of control and play. Nick looks a little bored although he is fine while he is actually playing himself. Amelia humours him by telling him she understands this is a little easy for him, but that it's great to have his help with the younger members of the group. This gives him permission to enjoy something he might feel he should be too old to take part in. Amelia wonders whether he has ever had much chance to be 'little' and play. When it comes to Arthur's turn, he tries to play the drum in unconventional ways, with his elbows, on the chair and on the floor. He seems to have a creative streak at the same time as watching Amelia and Susan carefully to see how far he will be allowed to go. Amelia stops him from hitting his head with the drum, but makes a feature of copying his new ideas which all the children enjoy. Philippa, however, is eager to please and do the right thing. She is a little put out when the children don't copy her rhythms exactly. Amelia purposely makes errors herself and then says that she sometimes finds it hard to copy unexpected playing. Amelia tries to acknowledge her need for perfection by commenting that different people find different things easy and hard, but that getting things right matters more to some people than to others.

After each of the children has had a turn on the drum, Amelia suggests that everyone should shut their eyes, and that as it is Patrick's last group he should put surprise instruments under each of the chairs. Once the instruments have been distributed Amelia plays a rhythmic piece on the piano, turning to the group as she plays and indicating that the group should play together.

Everyone joins in with the playing, drawn together by the beat and the predictable phrasing of the improvisation. Amelia suddenly drops the dynamic and slows down; everyone follows, but Patrick is the first to rebel, playing his bongo drums noisily. Amelia matches his loud playing and plays as loudly as she can for a few seconds before bringing the piece to a close. As soon as Amelia has finished playing she bends down and moves her hands slowly and carefully towards the floor, physically modelling what she would like the children to do, which is to put their instrument under their chair very quietly. Philippa puts her bells down very quietly, telling the group she hasn't made any noise, while Arthur gets us all to watch him very carefully putting the ocean drum under his chair. This is very difficult and he gets frustrated when the beads move around inside the drum. He starts again and Patrick purposely jogs him to make him make a noise. Amelia says 'Hold on, Patrick, don't make it harder for him,' consciously keeping her tone playful rather than confrontational. Susan turns to Nick, who is looking a little bored and says 'You had a special technique, last week, Nick, for putting the ocean drum down...can you show Arthur what you did?' Nick goes over to Arthur, tips the ocean drum up and shows him how to put it down so the beads remain still. In this way Susan successfully diverts Arthur from becoming frustrated while at the same time engaging Nick who was losing interest. Arthur follows Nick's instructions successfully and the whole group claps. Amelia immediately starts playing the piano again, this time incorporating one of Patrick's favourite tunes, the theme from EastEnders. Patrick immediately shouts out 'EastEnders' and Amelia smiles at him, mouthing 'Well done' as she continues playing. Arthur then suggests that his favourite tune, which is the theme to SpongeBob SquarePants, should be played. Amelia plays it on the piano and the children all start singing. Amelia winks at Nick, indicating to him that she appreciates the fact that he is willing to join in this 'young activity'. He grins, he seems to be enjoying himself. Arthur shouts and gets cross because Amelia hasn't got the words quite right. Amelia apologises and tells him that she doesn't know this song very well, can he tell her what the words are? He tries, but gets in a muddle. David, who has been joining in quietly in the background, comes to his rescue. The group tries again, and although Arthur insists that it's still not right, he accepts this version.

After the group music making a conducting game is suggested where three small percussion instruments are placed on the floor inside the circle of chairs. One person is the conductor and indicates who should play which instrument by using eyes and movements but no voice. Amelia puts the three instruments down and starts by asking the children to look at her eyes. She models what the game is about by looking at Susan who follows her indications. She then looks at Philippa who quickly picks up her cues, and the game proceeds. David and Nick turn out to be excellent conductors, Arthur needs a little help to use his eyes and look at people, and Patrick gets impatient with the waiting and feels it is unfair when he is not chosen first. Philippa tends to choose the adults as her musicians; she doesn't feel the children respond correctly to her instructions.

Next the bells are passed around the group while Amelia plays the piano. When two specific notes are played at the top of the piano the bells change direction. Again Amelia models this activity through making sure the change of direction first occurs when Susan, or children who she expects will quickly know what is expected, have the bells. Amelia can modify the difficulty of recognition of the two notes by leaving gaps, slowing the tempo or making the music she plays more or less complex. As she improvises on the piano she watches the children, trying to gauge who needs a turn next and how difficult to make the game for each person. She brings this activity to a close quite quickly as they are running out of time and she feels the children need to move to the next thing.

The group finishes with a rap, a rhythmic rendition of the words 'now it's time to finish the music' while participants clap and tap their knees. Amelia reminds the group that it is Patrick's last week and therefore his last music group so they should all think of something they will remember about Patrick after he has gone. She starts off by saying that she will remember Patrick singing the EastEnders tune. David says he will remember playing pool with Patrick. Nick looks sullen and cross and appears unwilling to say anything. Amelia wonders whether endings are a difficult topic for him. While keeping the rhythm going, Susan suggests that Patrick might remember playing football with Nick, which Nick seems to accept. Arthur takes his time choosing what he wants to say and Amelia is on tenterhooks, expecting an insult...but he comes out with the fact that he will remember Patrick doing a header in the playground. Patrick smiles; he appears sad, but pleased that his peers are saying nice things about him. Philippa says she will remember Patrick's smile. Susan and Amelia cringe internally as she appears to be taking on an adult role again.

As the children line up to walk to the dining room, Amelia feels a sense of achievement that they have managed to keep them all in the room during the whole group. She is pleased that the children have been able to share some positive moments together and at times support one another. Susan and Amelia return to the music room without the children to review the group together. They discuss each child in turn, making notes which they will later share with the rest of the team in the weekly management meeting. These notes will also help them to plan the group music therapy session the following week.

Yoga group

High levels of anxiety and stress are very common in children using mental health services. Many of the children have little confidence in their ability to think clearly or to work things out. Some of these children may also be uncoordinated and have little awareness of their own bodies and may have received a diagnosis of developmental co-ordination disorder (DCD). Others may be tense and anxious. For these children it may be particularly helpful to enable them to become aware of their bodies and their senses. Through self-awareness and an enhanced sense of inner tranquillity, children will gradually rebuild confidence, strength and emotional awareness.

At the Croft, the yoga group is run by Mark, a member of the nursing team who has a special interest in yoga and has been on a number of courses specialising in yoga for children, including Calm for Kids, led by Christiane Kerr (1999, 2009). He has adapted this approach to the needs of the children at the Croft. With children, the concepts of yoga are accessed indirectly through art, story-telling, play and creative games. The fundamentals of yoga, including classical postures, breathing exercises and relaxation, are incorporated into these activities. The children are encouraged to be aware of their physical state and how it links to their emotional state. Once the children have practised this approach they have additional skills to use when they become stressed or anxious.

On this particular Tuesday the children play the humming bee game in their yoga group. Patrick stays outside the room while a die is hidden. When he returns the children and the adults hum loudly when he is near to the object and quietly when he is far away. David, who usually is quite withdrawn in groups, can take part without the attention being on him. As he takes deep breaths to hum, his body visibly relaxes and the tension that is usually there dissipates. When Patrick misses the hiding place by a few inches, David can't resist giggling with Nick. The humming is now loud and intense, the energy in the group is almost tangible, and the children and the adults are aware that they are all doing something together, communicating and interacting in unison.

Later in the group the children become explorers in the rainforest. They pretend to wade through the forest and sit on yoga mats to canoe through rivers. When animals are spotted the children take on different animal postures based on classical yoga poses, but rather than staying still in the pose the children are encouraged to move and make animal noises, while particular attention is given to the breathing connected to these noises. Arthur comes into his own in this game, becoming an excellent frog, leaping around the room and making convincing 'gribbet' sounds. Nick is at first a slightly uncontrolled and aggressive lion, but after he is reminded that the animals in this rainforest do not hurt each other, he is able to put his energies into roaring loudly and concentrating on breathing appropriately to do this. This focused roaring seems to enable Nick to release some of his feelings of aggression.

The group finishes with a game of sleeping lions: the children are encouraged to lie on their backs with their heads resting on another child's abdomen. They are invited to close their eyes and try to be aware of both their own and their partner's breathing. Nick is unwilling to put his head on another child but agrees to put his head on a pillow that is on a member of staff's body. Arthur needs help to focus on the breathing and not jump up, but manages to lie down for a few minutes. Mark guides the relaxation by helping the children to imagine they are sleeping in the rainforest. There is a calm feeling in the room. At the end of the activity the children 'wake' and sit for a moment or two before leaving the room.

Playtime: outside and inside

Traditionally children look forward to breaktimes during their school day. Breaktimes are the unstructured periods of the day when children can choose activities and choose who to play with. Playtime traditionally is a release from work and expectation of achievement. However, for children with emotional, behavioural or developmental disorders, breaktime may present real challenges – they may not have any friends to play with and may find themselves the brunt of teasing and bullying, with no adults near at hand to help. They may struggle to understand the rules of the games or to play games with high levels of physical skill. Many children with special needs also find the transitions from structured adult-led activities to breaktime and back again hard to adjust to.

Within the inpatient programme, breaks are seen as therapeutic opportunities. They allow children to take a break from cognitive effort, they provide an opportunity for exercise, fresh air and fun, and they offer an opportunity to develop negotiation and relationship-building skills.

> Kelly and Mark, both members of the nursing team, are aware of the transition issues as they collect the children from school and take them to the playground. They have made sure that Alan (another member of the nursing team) is already outside to monitor Philippa, and prevent her from over-exercising. They also know that they must keep a close eye on Nick who climbed over the fence the previous week, leading to a chase around the surrounding buildings. They hope to engage both Arthur and Patrick in a game of football, giving them some structure and building up positive interaction so that they can have an enjoyable experience. They plan to involve Nick as a kind of coach, helping him to feel responsible and good about himself.
>
> As the children come out of school there is a palpable excitement, which Kelly and Mark can sense. There is, as always, a keen competition about who will be first to line up to get out into the playground. The children are like greyhounds waiting to be unleashed for a race, with huge amounts of energy ready to be dispensed. Patrick is particularly on edge this week because it is his last week on the Croft. He trips Arthur up and roars with laughter. Mark reacts swiftly, stepping into the physical space between the

two boys, thus averting a fracas and any physical retaliation by Arthur. At the same time Kelly asks Patrick to apologise and quickly ushers the other children into the playground. Kelly and Mark are experienced at working together and face these kinds of challenges every day. They trust each other's judgement and experience, and automatically pick up each other's cues as to how to deal with each situation as it arises.

Outside in the playground Nick is enjoying the responsibility he has been given to help the younger boys to play football. Kelly and Mark relax a little, hoping that he will not attempt to climb over the fence today. Watching the four boys playing football together it is impossible to imagine that a few seconds earlier World War Three was narrowly averted. David peels off and goes to the swings. He is not unfriendly or confrontational but often seems to prefer his own company. Kelly notices that he seems to be chattering to himself. She goes over to the swing next to him and engages him in conversation by asking him whether he likes football. In this informal and relaxed setting he confides in her that he used to like it but was disappointed when he didn't get into his village team. He also tells her that his father was really disappointed when this happened and he, David, felt he had let his dad down. He appears wistful and sad.

Alan is in the sandpit with Philippa. When she first arrived at the unit she seemed stiff and uncomfortable about playing. She had said that the sandpit was for much younger children and she seemed worried about getting messy. Initially she preferred to chat to adults during playtime, mainly about herself and her pets. However, nine weeks later she is regularly to be found in the sandpit, allowing herself to play and be a child. Arthur comes to join her. He is eager to build a mountain using as much sand as possible. Gradually this mountain takes over Philippa's area of the sand. Alan can feel that she is irritated even though she appears calm and she takes on an adult role of helping Arthur with his mountain. Alan notices that she finds it easier to give up her child role and prefers to please adults. Arthur's mountain is now huge. With a gleam in his eye and obvious enjoyment, he takes a running leap and jumps onto his mountain. Sand goes all over Philippa and she doesn't react, calmly shaking it off and getting out of the sandpit, smiling at Alan in an adult and knowing way. Arthur looks at Alan for a reaction, saying he will rebuild the mountain in the afternoon. Alan smiles at him in a supporting way, sensing Arthur's need to build and destroy in a safe way without reprimand or repercussion.

Towards the end of playtime Mark tells the children that they have two more minutes before it will be time to line up, giving the children time to finish off what they are doing and preparing them for the next transition.

LEGO club

LEGO groups were originally devised for children with autism spectrum disorders to enable them to develop pro-social co-operative social skills (Legoff and Sherman 2005). Many children are naturally attracted by LEGO and it can be a prime motivator to draw children into play. Unlike other groups at the Croft, this group happens in the evening and is not compulsory. It functions like an after-school activity – not all children take part, only those who want to and who agree to the group rules. The LEGO group is seen as something special to aspire to and children will often be motivated to try to overcome difficulties and control their outbursts to gain access to the club.

The club lasts between one and two hours and is staffed by two or three members of the nursing team. Between four and six children can take part and like other groups the children are of mixed ages and abilities. The group has a pre-determined structure and set of rules. At the beginning of the group the specific rules of LEGO club are stated:

- Build things together.
- Do not put LEGO in your mouth.
- Take turns.
- Do not jump ahead.
- Keep pieces for each model separate.

The children soon learn that these rules are necessary for the group to run smoothly and for everyone to have fun.

The group is split up into groups of two or three with one member of staff allocated to each subgroup. Within each subgroup children and staff are given a specific role: a part-finder, an instruction reader/engineer and a builder. The roles rotate in turn until the model is completed. It is the interaction between the people with the different roles that is crucial to the therapeutic process in the LEGO group. The engineer gives the part-finder instructions regarding which part should be found. The engineer then tells the builder where to place this part. To prepare for this group staff have to sort out LEGO pieces into categories and make sure that individual pieces can be easily found.

> Patrick was keen to come to the LEGO club right from the beginning of the admission. On a couple of occasions early on he couldn't attend because of behavioural problems during the day, but this improved and he became a regular member of the group. Staff soon realised that he managed better when given relatively simple models to build and they usually worked with him closely to help him succeed in his model building. He was able to interact with the group at the end of the session by showing his model to the other children and explain how a particular lever moved. For Patrick the fact that in the group specific children had clear roles and responsibilities helped him to understand exactly what was expected of him. He was also able to feel pride in his achievement, both in making a model successfully and managing a sustained social interaction, which was not something that he often experienced.

> Nick was initially suspicious of the LEGO club, thinking it was for younger children and not 'cool'. However, it was clear that he had not had many opportunities to play as a younger child and staff encouraged him to consider trying the group as they felt he would benefit from having a chance to allow himself to be playful. Nick was initially offered the task of helping Arthur, but the hope was that once in the group he would allow himself to just enjoy himself and have fun.

> Arthur always loved the LEGO group and was very skilful at constructing complicated models from his own imagination. Whilst he often approached the group in his own individualistic way, he gradually learnt to accept taking on different roles, even ones that were not his favourites. His mother was delighted to see him playing co-operatively with other children without incident – a very rare event in his life previously.

Summary

This chapter has described a few of the wide range of groups provided for children at the Croft for the purpose of assessment, diagnosis and short-term treatment. The group programme aims to combine different experiences for the children, some verbal, some non-verbal, some more physical, some more intellectual. The predictability of the programme and the consistency of group rules provide containment. These groups mirror the social setting of a school day – allowing the children to practise transitions from one activity to another. Some of the groups are particularly aimed at tackling emotional and relationship difficulties and could also be adapted to different settings such as schools or residential homes. Some groups are more structured than others and some groups, such as the music group and the yoga group, require special expertise from the group leader. However, in all of the groups the key element is to have skilled sensitive adults who listen to the children, are attuned to their needs and creatively adapt the material to suit changing situations and circumstances.

Chapter 8

Understanding the Individual

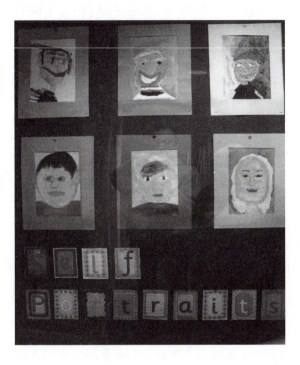

Children's views of themselves

Introduction

All mental health services are focused on understanding children as individuals as well as considering the impact of their environment on their development and functioning. When assessing children who are living in complex social situations, this becomes more challenging as their individual characteristics and views may be overshadowed by difficulties in their family functioning.

At the Croft, the child is admitted with other family members, and whilst this provides the opportunity to assess the child holistically in his family context, it also presents a real risk that the needs or views of the adults are prominent, and those of the individual child are pushed into the background. This risk has been illustrated in reviews of serious child abuse cases in the UK over the years. In Lord Laming's (2003) report into the death of a young girl called Victoria Climbié, amongst many other systems failures, he highlighted the lack of serious attempts to gain information directly from the child about her experiences and an over-reliance by professionals on accounts given by the girl's carers. Tragically in her case this led to her death, due to physical abuse and neglect.

Trying to unravel the complex interactions between inherent characteristics and socially determined patterns of behaviour is also a challenging task. In this situation there is a danger that any maladaptive behaviour in the child is ascribed to his environment and inherent problems such as learning difficulties or neuro-developmental disorders will be missed. This could lead to a failure to make provision for these needs.

To understand the individual child, the aim is to gain an in-depth understanding of the whole child including his personality, his developmental strengths and weaknesses, his beliefs and attitudes towards his difficulties, how he views his family and indeed how he perceives his treatment.

Not all children will have sufficiently well-developed language skills to be able to express themselves in words, but by using a variety of modalities and contexts the team obtains a rich variety of information about the child. This information has to be interpreted with an awareness of the constraints of an inpatient setting, the fact that the child may function somewhat differently in the unit setting than in his own home, school or community, and that the relatively short timeframe of an average admission (around six weeks) provides only a snapshot of the child's life. However, even taking these constraints into account, an intensive assessment in a contained setting with multiple therapeutic modalities is likely to produce the most comprehensive assessment available.

Although the distinction between assessment and treatment is not always clear, some of the assessments will involve an element of treatment. Therapeutic treatment or interventions can act as further assessment, helping to determine whether a particular child would benefit from a particular treatment on discharge. Sometimes children will have entered the unit having already experienced some form of individual therapy or protective relationship, and for a small proportion it could be ongoing. In the latter case the therapist has to consider the importance of ensuring that any ongoing work or relationships are not disrupted.

This chapter describes the various assessments and treatments that are available at the Croft. None of them are unique to the Croft, but carrying them out in the context of an inpatient admission may have both advantages and disadvantages or raise issues within the particular assessment or intervention. These issues are discussed within each section.

Co-ordinating the assessment

Before and during the admission the team will be thinking about which aspects should be included in the individual assessment. Each discipline will have its own framework for assessment which will be implemented either individually or in collaboration with other team members. Care is taken not to overload a child with assessments, to time interventions appropriately and not to repeat investigations unnecessarily.

The assessments and observations may also lead to new questions and further investigations, to a new approach or a new way of thinking about the child. For example, the nursing team may have concerns that a parent and child have particular attachment difficulties. This may then be explored further with the child in a story stem assessment (described later on pp.151–153). The story stem assessment might indicate the attachment patterns of the child but may also raise new issues regarding a child's anxieties about domestic violence, which might link to themes in the family therapy sessions or suggest a new issue to consider.

All the information gathered by the team on individual children is drawn together and discussed at weekly multi-disciplinary meetings. Throughout the admission, different theoretical perspectives will be considered and the collective findings will be integrated to create an agreed working hypothesis or formulation.

Different types of assessments are used: formal assessments, some of which are standardised, and informal assessments, which might overlap with short-term therapy. Both types are explored in this chapter.

Key worker system

In common with many other care systems, the Croft uses a key worker system. Key workers are nurses and health care assistants who provide the bulk of face-to-face care for a child and family. They work shifts throughout the day and night and will be observing and working with families directly. An example of their observations of daily living skills is given in Appendix 6. Their observations are crucial in keeping the individual child at the forefront of the assessment in the context of having the whole family and indeed many families at the Croft at one time. From the early assessment of suitability for admission, through the admission and through the discharge process, the key worker keeps the needs and desires of the child in mind and works as an advocate for the child.

Because the Croft is an inpatient unit the nursing team work in shifts and therefore the child has a key worker team which includes three or four members of staff. This ensures that on each shift there will be a key worker who has a detailed knowledge of each child. The integrated team approach to each child (described in Chapter 2) enables detailed observations of the child to be cross-referenced. For example, the team might be interested in tracking the child's levels of impulsivity in different situations, and with different people. In addition, as referred to in Chapter 3, this allows the team to support each other, which can be very important with children with complex difficulties. It also allows multiple perspectives on the child's behaviour, adding up to a more thorough picture of the child's difficulties.

Another advantage of having a number of key people working with the child is that the child's relationships with adults can be observed. For example, a child with a history of neglect or abuse will often make very intense, emotionally dependent relationships with their key workers whilst a child with an autism spectrum disorder would be much more likely to show a similar pattern of behaviour with all staff.

The key worker has a crucial role in co-ordinating the care plan for each child and this will include updating other professionals about the child's day-to-day progress and providing advice on how to approach the child. The key worker spends a lot of time with the child, especially in the early part of the admission, observing the child and getting to know him. For example, key workers can report on the child's use of and understanding of language, on patterns of behaviour that might affect other assessments and even on rewards and consequences that work for the child.

> Nick was very difficult to engage. He was reluctant to see any therapists on his own and trying to undertake structured assessments had not worked well. One of Nick's key workers had noticed that Nick's behaviour often escalated before a session if he knew that it was imminent. They guessed that Nick was getting anxious about the sessions although he was unable to voice that himself. They also noted that Nick was very slow to get started in the morning, but also got tired and more irritable later on in the afternoon. It was therefore suggested that assessments might work best in the middle of the day.
>
> Nick was immune to sanctions, but he would work towards rewards such as playing football with his favourite member of staff or having a later bedtime. He also loved motorbikes and would chat easily about them. This information helped the team members work out when and, to a certain extent, how to do their assessments. The psychiatrist managed to get hold of a motorbike magazine with stickers and used this as an incentive for Nick to have a session, with her assessing his mental state and the impact of previous traumatic experiences. The music therapist timed her sessions in the middle of the day and linked attendance at the sessions with football sessions afterwards.

As well as the more informal work, the key workers also provide the child with structured, but flexible, individual sessions. The content of these sessions is linked to the care plan and admission aims, so, for example, for a child with an eating disorder triggered by bullying at school the sessions might encompass discussions both about healthy eating and on coping with social difficulties.

Early in the admission the child will work with the key worker using the key worker book (for an example of a key worker book see Appendix 7). This is a series of structured worksheets that the key worker uses to get to know the child. It includes his likes and dislikes, his understanding of why he is at the Croft, thoughts and feelings about friends and family and what he feels he is good or bad at. The book introduces the child to individual sessions gently, and helps the child to begin to feel relaxed in staff company. One helpful element to aid attendance at the session is to give the child the choice of what game to play at the end of the session. This also serves to end the session on a relaxed, happy, neutral activity. For some children with attention problems the book might take a few sessions to complete. For other children, even these low-key flexible sessions might be too challenging and a more subtle approach to individual time is needed.

> At the beginning of Nick's second week one of his key workers suggested an individual session to look at the key worker book. Nick was anxious and irritable before the session, swearing at adults and saying the session was boring even before it had begun. As soon as the key worker showed him the book he started kicking chairs and overturning furniture and the session had to be halted. The key worker team discussed this in the weekly group supervision meeting. The team decided to try a different approach. Nick had started to develop a positive relationship with a male nurse who owned a much loved Harley Davidson motorbike. It was agreed that Nick and the nurse would have some sessions making a model motorbike together. This gave the nurse a chance to chat informally with Nick, as he did so including a number of the topics that appeared in the key worker book. He discovered that Nick thought that he had no good features and that the only thing he was good at was annoying people. Nick also talked about his mother's boyfriends, describing their motorbikes, their use of alcohol and drugs and which ones hit him and his mum. Nick's key worker tried to suggest strategies that Nick could use to manage his angry feelings but Nick wasn't able to take any of these on board due to the ongoing uncertainty about his future with his mother.

Alongside the key worker book other structured activities are used. For example, key workers regularly use the *All About Me Game* (Hemmings 2003). This game encourages the child to answer questions about themselves in a fun context, it provides the opportunity to explore the child's world but because the child and the key worker take turns to answer questions, it is less intimidating than a more formal questioning approach. For other children having sessions of craft or LEGO building may be the best setting for conversation.

David was quite happy to work through the key worker book in week one but he resolutely refused to talk about his anxiety, or his experience of hearing threatening voices. In week two they played the *All About Me Game* and this did stimulate David to talk about his fears and in particular his fear that he was going mad. He and his key worker talked about ways he could cope with stress and worry. In week three David had a lot of other assessments going on, and therefore did not have an individual session, as the team knew by then he would find this too difficult and didn't want to overload him. However, in the evenings he often sought out his key worker to play LEGO or have a game of pool.

There was a team discussion about whether David should have some sessions with the psychologist to look at ways of coping with his anxiety, but the team decided that since David already had a good relationship with his key worker, it would be best to capitalise on this, and the psychologist offered to supervise the key worker sessions and advise on some anxiety management work. In week four David and his key worker reviewed the coping strategies they had discussed in week two. David said that understanding that the voices were linked to his anxiety had helped him feel better. They started working on anxiety management. During the next couple of sessions they talked about what made him anxious, and how to solve the problems caused by anxiety-provoking situations. They worked on his self-esteem using positive feedback and re-framing negatives, for example, pointing out to David that although he felt his strategies had failed as he was still hearing voices, the voices had actually significantly reduced in frequency as had the degree to which they were interfering with his daily life. In David's final week he finished his key worker booklet, and revisited the strategies he had learnt and he and his key worker talked about how he would handle leaving the unit and going back to school.

One of the roles of the key worker is to collate all the detailed observations made by the nursing team during the week. A system of documenting has been developed to enable key information regarding specific diagnoses to be collated methodically and easily. This methodical approach ensures that the strengths as well as the difficulties are recorded, and stops an over-emphasis on particularly traumatic moments. It also ensures that the team do not become over-focused on seeking to support a specific diagnosis, but remain curious and open. A copy of this document is included in Appendix 8.

Key workers may be asked by members of the team to make observations focused on a specific question. For example, a clinical psychologist assessing a child's cognitive ability may ask one of the nursing team to observe how well a child plans ahead when playing a game of Connect Four with a younger sibling.

Feedback to parents

An important part of understanding and interpreting the observations that the team make of a child is including the views of the parents. This enables staff to compare their perceptions and interpretations of observations with that of the parent. This is done through everyday, in-the-moment conversations, and also by encouraging parents to read the nursing observation sheets at the end of each week. Parents may do this with a key worker or on their own, but they are encouraged to add their own views to the records if they wish to. Parents often say that reading the nursing observations helps them to understand how the team are seeing their child, and conversations arising from this are often very fruitful. Looking at areas of convergence and divergence helps both the team and the parent reflect on their perceptions and can assist in forming a consensual understanding of what may be driving a particular pattern of behaviour or emotional response.

Formal assessments

If a child has come to the Croft it is almost certain that his difficulties are complex. For example, Nick had a diagnosis of attention deficit hyperactivity disorder (ADHD) and had been excluded from school for antisocial behaviour. His mother reported that he had a terrible memory, and this was often seen when given instructions. It was not certain whether he could not retain instructions because he did not understand them, or whether he did not remember them, or whether he just did not want to follow them. A formal assessment of Nick's needs could help start to answer this question.

At the Croft a number of structured formal assessments are available, including neuropsychology assessment, use of questionnaires, the Smart Cat educational assessment, the Autism Diagnostic Observation Schedule (ADOS), story stem assessments and a diagnostic assessment using music therapy. All of these are embedded in the overall assessment and are used together to produce a picture of the child's strengths and weaknesses.

Neuropsychological assessment

Arthur, who was six at the time of admission, had a diagnosis of ADHD and a speech impediment, but Arthur's parents and other professionals working with him wondered whether he also had an autism spectrum disorder. During Arthur's stay at the Croft there were parts of the programme Arthur seemed to manage well and he gave an impression of some ability, whereas at other times he appeared not to understand at all. His mother had reported that he had a 'phenomenal memory' and could draw maps from memory, and had apparently learnt to read very early. However, neither she, nor Arthur's teacher, were sure if he understood what he read.

Reports from his school indicated that formal assessment had not been possible due to his reluctance to be tested and generally oppositional and destructive behaviour. The local education authority were undertaking an educational assessment to try to establish how much support he needed in school and a detailed assessment of his learning profile would help to establish his specific needs.

Children who have lost confidence in themselves and in adults will require a great deal of nurturing to regain the sense that they can tackle new challenges. The individualised, contained environment of the Croft gives the child an opportunity to re-engage with both group and individual activities. Rather than feeling singled out by individual attention children will see their peers also taking part in one-to-one assessments. Testing can be done over several sessions with plenty of breaks. If children cannot manage on one occasion, they can return to the group programme and be seen another day. Some children cannot tolerate any change to their routine, so the clinician may need to come to them, and undertake the assessment in a corner of the classroom.

The aim is to give the child the best chance of demonstrating his optimum level. At the same time, recommendations also need to take into account that the child's actual level of functioning or performance may be lower in more everyday circumstances, for example in a busy mainstream classroom environment.

The assessment itself gives an opportunity to observe the child in a standardised clinical situation (Anderson *et al.* 2001). During the testing process a number of clinical observations are made that complement the testing results. These include children's attitude to being assessed, their level of arousal, their attention skills, including their ability to shift their attention, their sense of confidence, sensory impairments, executive control, visual scanning strategies, laterality, motor skills, learning style, social interaction, use of eye contact to communicate, and so on. The tests used in the unit include the Wechsler Intelligence Scale for Children (WISC IV) (Wechsler 2003), which taps a number of cognitive skills including verbal reasoning, perceptual reasoning and working memory (processes used for temporarily storing and manipulating information). Although the WISC, in common with other neuropsychological tests, must be scored and administered in a standardised way, it is essential to also take into consideration children with special needs and be somewhat flexible in order to allow them to demonstrate their abilities.

Often children with complex neuro-developmental and emotional disorders show a scatter of scores even within one type of ability, for example, verbal ability (Humphrey 2006). Particular patterns can be seen in different conditions, for example children with autism spectrum difficulties often have significant discrepancies between their verbal and non-verbal scores. They may also perform in the above average range in subtests which tap into skills such as visuo-spatial manipulation (Edgin and Pennington 2005). Therefore looking at individual tests or even individual answers to questions can be helpful in understanding the child's profile.

Tests of attainment are also used to identify discrepancies between a child's intellectual functioning and his achievement in spelling, reading or mathematics. Such a discrepancy would suggest a specific learning difficulty in the corresponding academic area. Specific learning difficulties, especially in the area of literacy, are common and can contribute to emotional and behavioural problems.

They are often found alongside ADHD, language disorders and autism spectrum disorders to name but a few (Cantwell 1991; Willicut and Pennington 2000).

Another test that is used is the Behavioural Assessment of Dysexecutive Syndrome for Children (BADS-C; see Emslie *et al.* 2003). This measures aspects of executive function. The term 'executive function' describes a set of cognitive abilities that control and regulate other abilities and behaviours. Executive functions are necessary for goal-directed behaviour: they include the ability to start and stop actions, to monitor and change behaviour as needed, to plan future behaviour when faced with novel tasks and situations and to allow individuals to anticipate outcomes and adapt to changing situations. Executive function is often dysfunctional in many childhood psychological disorders (Pennington and Ozonoff 1996).

Other reasons for carrying out neuropsychological assessments include providing a baseline measurement so that future progress can be monitored. They can also be used as a vehicle to help parents understand some of their child's difficulties, to increase their tolerance towards difficult behaviour and to give alternative strategies to work with their children.

> In Arthur's case, neuropsychological assessment wasn't even attempted until his fifth week at the Croft. By this time he was familiar with the psychologist and willing to come to the session with the promise of a chance to look at some maps on the wall in the assessment room. It was decided to start with the WISC to give an initial idea of his learning level.
>
> In order start the session positively Arthur was offered some felt tip pens and paper to 'draw whatever he wanted'. He chose to draw a map and was happy to tell the psychologist all about it, in a rather long and rambling manner and with little reference to whether she was listening.
>
> The psychologist was aware from previous observations of Arthur in the Croft that he found it difficult to carry out instructions that were not on his terms. In order therefore to move Arthur onto the first subtest (block design), the box containing the bricks was shown to him, and he was sufficiently curious to see its contents that it was possible to move him smoothly into starting the subtest.

The task required Arthur to replicate a set of modelled or printed two-dimensional geometric patterns using red and white blocks within a specified time limit. However, it was immediately evident that he wanted to set the agenda and carry out the task in the way he preferred, that is, to make patterns of his own choosing.

In order to keep Arthur engaged the psychologist allowed him to make his chosen pattern, before moving on to the next presented design. Fortunately Arthur accepted the next design and in fact the test was sufficiently intrinsically rewarding to be able to complete the subtest without resorting to letting him do his own design again.

During the first session it was possible to carry out six of the subtests of the WISC. Once he had settled into the session, Arthur almost seemed to enjoy the structure and clear rules of the assessment.

Arthur scored well on some subtests and poorly on others, but did not show a consistent pattern. Because he did have an unusual pattern of scores, as well as looking at his scores in comparison to children of his own age, the psychologist looked at individual answers to questions and also his pattern of replies. For example Arthur's typical replies were 'Don't you know!' or 'Why are you asking?' Arthur also struggled with questions involving social understanding. This gave an important insight into how Arthur might struggle with school and suggested that he had a similar profile to children on the autistic spectrum.

In Arthur's case, the answers he gave and how he approached the tasks suggested that it might be helpful to look at his executive functioning. He had difficulties with transitions between activities and did not respond well to novel tasks and situations. He also struggled to stop activities he was enjoying. A number of things could explain this, including having an autistic spectrum disorder, having problems with his executive functions or perhaps being 'difficult' and deciding he just didn't want to do the next task when asked.

The psychologist administered the BADS-C and was surprised to find that Arthur managed all the subtests well within the normal range so it seemed that executive dyscontrol did not account for his struggles with transitions. The psychologist decided to ask the key workers to undertake focused observations of Arthur during transitions to establish if there was a pattern.

Assessing social communication

Many children who come to this service have very poor social skills, as referred to in the previous chapter. Typically they find it very hard to initiate and maintain a reciprocal conversation, share or take turns. They tend to see the world only in relation to their own needs and some can find it hard to notice and understand the emotional responses of others to their behaviour. When these social interaction problems exist alongside high levels of impulsivity and poor emotional regulation then children often display very antisocial behaviour. In this situation one question that is often asked is whether these difficulties relate to inherent (probably inherited) biological traits (such as autism spectrum disorders) or whether they have been caused by inadequate or interrupted care and nurturing, particularly in early infancy (attachment disorders).

So how does one go about distinguishing these two types of problem that can manifest themselves in similar and overlapping ways?

Getting as full a picture of children's development and the environment they are growing up in will give strong clues. Usually children with autistic spectrum disorder will show significant delays in their development of language and motor skills alongside a tendency to repetitive and stereotyped behaviour (Baron-Cohen 2008). Children with attachment problems on the other hand show more problems in the areas of emotional regulation (Cassidy 1994) and stability of relationships. However, both groups of children may often have very great difficulty in relating to peers and adults and they often have sleeping, eating and toileting problems too.

Using structured assessments to examine both these areas can be very helpful. The Autism Diagnostic Interview (ADI; see Lord, Rutter and LaCouteur 1994) is used to obtain detailed information about development in the areas of communication, social interaction and any history of repetitive behaviours. Obtaining information from parents about problems in their relationship and care of their children in their infant years can be more difficult as, understandably, parents are eager to describe themselves as loving, caring parents and are resistant to thinking that any aspect of their care-giving may have damaged their child. In this area it is important to try to obtain information from health visitors or nurseries that may have very important observations of the parent–child interaction.

Generally, direct observation of children in a variety of settings can help to show particular patterns of interaction and triggers for disturbance; for example, children with attachment disorders often show an intensification of their difficulties when they are separated from or reunited with their caregivers whilst children with autism spectrum disorders often show more difficulty when their general day-to-day routine is changed.

Direct standardised assessments of children can also add useful information to the overall picture. The ADOS (Lord *et al.* 1989) is used to look for signs of autism, and an assessment called story stem assessments (Hodges *et al.* 2003) looks at how children think about family relationships and attachment issues.

Autism Diagnostic Observation Schedule (ADOS)

This assessment was designed by Lord and colleagues (1989) and consists of a number of activities (about 12 to 13) that are done with a child over a 30- to 45-minute session. The aim is to make the session as fun and informal as possible and it is designed to encourage social interaction and communication. This includes tasks such as asking a child to make up a story for three characters and for the assessor to join in the play and to introduce new ideas into the play. This enables the assessor to determine if the child can imagine and integrate other ideas into his play or whether he becomes very fixed on his own agenda to the exclusion of other people. Typically, primary-age children love to play with others, especially adults, and love it when adults are playing on their level. Children with autism spectrum disorders, on the other hand, either find it difficult to do any imaginary play or, if they can, often have a very fixed idea of how the play should be and cannot be flexible to allow new ideas into their stories.

Other tasks include asking the child to mime an everyday action, to read a story from a picture book and to answer questions about his emotions and friendships. Children's responses are then coded in the areas of communication and social interaction and there are cut-off scores for autism and autism spectrum disorders.

Using a combination of the information from the ADI, scores from the ADOS and direct observation of a child in a number of situations, both structured and unstructured, one can usually be clear as to whether a child's difficulties would fit into the pattern shown by people with autism spectrum disorders.

Arthur's ADOS assessment

Arthur was, as usual, reluctant to come to the assessment session. He hated any change to his ordinary daily routine and said he wanted to stay with the other children in the art group – however, after some gentle persuasion and the psychiatrist showing him a map of the London Underground in her diary, he agreed to come. They started the sessions talking about maps – the psychiatrist tried to introduce other topics but Arthur skilfully turned the conversation back to maps or countries each time. Arthur managed to do a puzzle but when he found that he had not enough pieces to complete the puzzle he just stopped, without asking for help. He refused to even attempt making up a story with characters but became fascinated with a spinning holographic toy instead, becoming very engrossed. He became very restless when the assessment became more talk-based – when asked to say why people got married he said 'to continue the species'. Generally his speech was rather formal for a child of his age, and his eye contact was fleeting. He spoke only in response to questions, and he only became more interested in communicating when there was any mention of his favourite subjects. Generally the psychiatrist was left feeling that Arthur didn't care whether she was in the room or not.

Story stem assessments

This assessment has been developed by Jill Hodges and colleagues at the Anna Freud Centre in London and also incorporates some stories from the McCarthy battery used in the USA (Bretherton *et al.* 1990). The aim of the assessment is to tap into how the child thinks about family relationships as reflected in his imagination and play with family figures. The child is given a family of four play people, a father, mother and two siblings of the same gender as the child being assessed. The assessor then starts by setting up a scenario for the family and asking the child to finish the story in whatever way he would want to. There are 13 scenarios which have been developed to access the child's attachment system – the scenarios have some dilemma or difficulty in relationships and the assessor then notes down how the child deals with this dilemma in their play. So, for instance, one scenario would be a child spilling a jug of juice whilst the family are sitting down waiting to eat a meal, another is a child witnessing parents arguing about lost keys, another involves a child being injured after ignoring the parents' instructions to take care.

Children with attachment disorders may show particular patterns in their representations of family relationships – there may be an anxious response whereby any problem is immediately resolved or denied, or they may show an ambivalent response in which parental figures are variably idolised or denigrated.

Any information gathered during this assessment has to be understood in the context of observations of the child and his parents and the history of the family; it should not be thought of as a direct replaying of actual events but as an insight into the child's view of the way families operate.

Patrick's story stem assessment

The psychologist had set out a table with the play figures and dolls' house furniture ready and when Patrick walked through the door he was immediately drawn to the toys. The psychologist explained to Patrick that she was going to start some stories and he could finish them however he wanted. First Patrick picked out names for the two boys in the family – he called them Alex and Paul – and then the psychologist set the scene for the first story. In the story the children and their dad are sitting at the kitchen table as the mum is preparing dinner. Paul is thirsty and he leans over the table to get a jug of juice but it falls out of his hands onto the floor. The psychologist then sits back to let Patrick complete the story – he sits looking at the figures for a few seconds, then he grabs the dad and shouts: 'You stupid, stupid boy – why did you do that? – you are killing me,' and then Patrick picks up the dad and uses him to kick at Paul. He then picks up Alex and makes the figure fly around the room, saying 'He is superman' – the Alex figure then dive-bombs the dad figure sending him flying off the table – then he attacks the mum and she joins dad on the floor. Patrick then picks up both boys and they fly around together – 'Let's go to Disneyland,' they say. Patrick then transforms the dolls' house furniture into Disney characters that come up to the boys and they each say 'Welcome to the Magic Kingdom' in turn.

Patrick continued with another six stories. At the end the psychologist reviewed her transcripts of the stories and noted down how the family figures were depicted and the themes of interactions. She noted that there was very little emotional warmth or care shown to the children by the adults, and there was a very high level of negative emotion between the children and the parents. The children seemed to derive emotional support from each other and they were either depicted as very powerful, as in the story about the spilt juice, or as victims. Stories sometimes had a fantastical, magical ending or ended abruptly with unresolved conflict or distress.

When the psychologist fed back the results to the rest of the team they discussed how this fitted into other information, such as Patrick's very volatile relationships with both his parents and staff and his very low self-esteem.

Music therapy diagnostic assessments (MTDAs)

The music therapy diagnostic assessments (MTDAs) were developed at the Croft in order to assist the team with the diagnosis of the children's strengths and difficulties. In the Friday morning management meetings it was often apparent that the music therapist had noticed very different aspects of the children's behaviours from the rest of the team, indicating that the MTDAs were serving a different purpose from other assessments. Between 2000 and 2004 a research investigation was carried out at the Croft to compare MTDA results with ADOS results (Oldfield 2004). Over a period of two years 30 children suspected of being on the autistic spectrum had ADOS and MTDA assessments. The two assessments showed 72 per cent of agreement between diagnostic categories (autism, borderline autism and no autism); however, they also showed significant differences in scores of individual questions. For example, the MTDA was less likely to consider the children's social overtures to be on the autistic spectrum, but more likely to score autistic spectrum-type behaviours when looking at the children's ritualistic behaviours. This showed that the MTDA could serve a useful and distinct purpose in helping the psychiatric team to diagnose children with autism.

The MTDA consists of two half-hour sessions which usually occur at the same time on two consecutive weeks. Children are invited to choose instruments to play from a wide range of percussion instruments including a drum kit, piano, electric keyboard and smaller percussion instruments such as bongo drums. The music therapist often engages the child in free, non-verbal improvisation and dialogues, but may also encourage the child to make up songs, learn short pieces, or generally explore the instruments. It is through the child's involvement in the music making that strengths and difficulties will be observed and assessed (Oldfield 2006).

A scoring sheet from the MTDA is included in Appendix 9. One very helpful aspect of the MTDA is its ability to engage and assess non-verbal communication in some children who find any verbally based assessment too challenging. Often children with specific language difficulties show much better social interaction skills in the MTDA than in the ADOS.

Arthur's MTDA

When the music therapist, Amelia, went to collect Arthur from school for his second MTDA session, he was ready to come, having been reminded earlier in the morning meeting that this session was taking place. On the way to the music room he told Amelia that he had made a map of the Croft the previous evening and knew exactly where the music room was. He also told her that he wanted to play the drum kit because he was good at drumming. Amelia responded by saying that she was looking forward to his drum kit playing; she had enjoyed it the previous week.

Once in the music room, Amelia told Arthur that she would start with a 'Hello song' on the guitar, as she had done the previous week. Arthur sat down in a grumpy way saying he wanted the drum kit straight away. As soon as the song started he relaxed and smiled, said 'I know that one' and asked Amelia to sing it again.

Later in the session, as Amelia improvised on the piano to accompany Arthur's drumming, she marvelled at how free and at ease he seemed to be while playing the drum kit. She tried copying his rhythmic suggestions which provoked a smile and seemed to make Arthur feel good about his playing. She also tried mismatching and playing different rhythms. This sometimes caused Arthur to look up and change his own playing to copy Amelia's but, at other times, particularly when her playing was very different to his, he seemed oblivious of her, continuing with whatever rhythmic pattern he had initiated. The duet went on for over five minutes and they came to a common ending, both feeling pleased with the shared musical experience.

After the drumming, Arthur chose the bass xylophone for himself and the metallophone for Amelia. Together they made up a story/song, accompanying the words with instrumental playing. Arthur decided the story should be about two dogs that went to the park to play. When Amelia continued by saying that there was a crocodile under the slide, Arthur did not look pleased. He said: 'if I'd known there was going to be a crocodile…I would have made them big dogs…'

Towards the end of the session Amelia suggested that they both play kazoos. Arthur immediately started singing a well-known nursery rhyme into the kazoo. Amelia tried to draw him into a kazoo sound exchange by making a variety of responses to his singing. She tried sounding surprised, angry and frightened. However, Arthur could not be drawn into a kazoo exchange; instead he kept coming back to his favourite SpongeBob SquarePants television song, playing and singing but not responding interactively in any way to Amelia's reactions. Amelia eventually joined him, supporting and accompanying his song. This prompted Arthur to suggest that they make a recording of the song that Amelia agreed to arrange for the following week.

When Amelia reviewed the session and scored the MTDA, she realised that Arthur presented a mixed picture. On the one hand, he appeared to be flexible, communicative and creative when engaged in musical interactions while playing the drums. On the other hand, he liked to be the initiator and only sometimes responded to Amelia's musical suggestions. In the kazoo exchanges he was particularly uncommunicative, perhaps because this was closer to speech than non-verbal musical exchanges. On the MTDA he scored for borderline autism, but not for classical autism.

In addition to these direct assessments, questionnaires can provide a standardised approach to gathering information about children. Many of these, such as the Child Behaviour Checklist (Achenbach and Rescorla 2001), are designed to be completed by a number of respondents and have parent, teacher and youth versions. The Conners assessments of ADHD symptoms (Conners 1997) also seek views from parents and teachers. Many of the measures that ask the children themselves about their difficulties are designed for children aged 11 and over. At the Croft, even if the child's chronological age is 11, his emotional or cognitive age might not be, and the questionnaire might not yield a useful result. Often the information needed can be gained less formally, using the strategies described elsewhere in this chapter.

Individual therapy at the Croft

Whilst individual assessment at the Croft can benefit from the multiplicity of information and observations, the short-term nature of most admissions means that undertaking individual therapy can be more challenging. Often a very important task is to establish what mode of individual work is suitable for a child so that this can inform the ongoing plan for the child after discharge. It may also be that there are short-term goals that can be worked on and often it can be that the process of assessment is therapeutic in itself. For example, it was described above how David used individual time to understand and feel more mastery over his voices. This was the first time he had been able to do this and even the process of talking about his voices made them less scary and helped the team identify anxiety as his key issue.

Because of the time-limited nature of Croft admissions termination issues have to be addressed very early in the assessment/therapy process, and because of team working it is also very important to address the issue of therapeutic confidentiality. In order to get as comprehensive and accurate a picture of the child as possible, much of the information gained from the child and family is shared with the whole Croft team as well as the referring professionals. This also means that usually the themes that the child discusses in individual sessions, including therapy sessions, are shared with the parents. Issues around sharing information need to be addressed with the child early on in sessions, and often the child is involved in deciding how, what and when information is shared with the parents. For example, initially Philippa did not want to share her therapy sessions with her mother. However, as they progressed, Philippa realised that her mum probably did know a lot of the things she was saying anyway and eventually she was happy to have a joint session to share information.

A number of different therapy modalities are commonly available at the Croft and they complement each other in their approach. These include cognitive behaviour therapy (CBT), play therapy and music therapy.

Cognitive behaviour therapy (CBT)

CBT is an approach that encompasses both behaviour therapy, using strategies to reward positive behaviour and reduce negative behaviours, and cognitive strategies to challenge dysfunctional thought patterns and related behaviours. The former is used extensively throughout the Croft programme to help parents and staff manage challenging behaviours. The latter approach is used individually with some children. There is research evidence to support its use with children with eating difficulties, obsessive compulsive problems and anxiety disorders (Cottrell *et al.* 2005). CBT can also be useful with other difficulties but it does require a certain level of cognitive functioning. These children are the ones who can see associations between how they are feeling and thinking and the impact this has on their behaviour. Therefore it might be appropriate to offer this kind of therapy to children who are failing to manage their anger or struggling to get to sleep due to anxiety.

When children arrive at the Croft they are expected to take part in various activities. These include going to the school and taking part in the group programme, which includes art and music groups, and engaging with other therapies, such as family therapy. CBT is a little different to this, as it relies on the child being willing to engage with the therapist. Individual structured therapy is often quite verbal, although creative strategies are widely used throughout engagement and intervention. It is also more directly about the child's stated difficulties than the creative therapies. Therefore the child has to have some motivation to talk about his difficulties.

Starting CBT with Philippa

After eight weeks at the Croft, Philippa had just started talking about her worries about being fat and being accepted when she went back to school. Prior to this she had denied any thoughts of being fat and talked about being full and just not feeling like eating. Although both her parents wanted her to have individual therapy from early in the admission, she found talking about her eating very difficult and would not say much apart from 'I don't know.' By week eight, Philippa was talking more openly about her fears about eating with her key worker and when asked whether she wanted to have some help with her thoughts, she admitted she was willing to try it.

Because of the age of the children and the short-term nature of their admission to the Croft it may be difficult for them to access CBT. For some, such as Philippa, it is possible to wait until they feel ready to start some therapy.

For most children the engagement process is the key to therapy. Engagement at the Croft utilises the same strategies as anywhere else. It is important to start with the child's agenda and think about what the child wants help with (Friedberg and McClure 2002). This may or may not fit in with the agenda of the family and the referrer. Therapy also needs to fit in with the overall admission plan.

There are also aspects of being in intensive multi-modal treatment which make this process easier. It is easier to establish the initial rapport with the child as the therapist will know a lot about his day-to-day activity. Also having already met the family it can be easier to talk about family issues as they arise. Furthermore, the children will be used to talking regularly about their emotions and feelings, and therefore can be primed to use a therapeutic talking approach.

> David had started talking about his voices to his key worker and this had made them seem less scary, but the team thought he may benefit from a CBT approach and in week three he met with the therapist. David was very clear about what he wanted help with. He was beginning to make links with what had happened to him in the past and what was happening in his head now, but it still scared him a great deal. The psychiatrist was hoping for additional information to identify whether he was suffering from post-traumatic stress disorder (PTSD), his parents were keen to stop his aggression, and his school were hoping that someone would help reverse the recent decline in his learning. However, the initial sessions were kept short and regular, and they focused on David telling the therapist about what he was currently finding difficult. This then helped his key worker complement the work using anxiety management techniques.

There are frequent opportunities at the Croft to work with other team members to ensure that the work being done is relevant to the overall care plan. Sometimes children will have conversations with their key worker that are not the same as the conversations they have with the therapist. Sometimes the same conversation is played out again and again. This is very useful information about the child's inner world, and also allows the team to make decisions about who could be the most helpful team member for the child.

Some children's parents, like Philippa's, are desperate for their child to have therapy as they see this as very important in their child's recovery. Sometimes it is the children themselves who want the therapy. In outpatient settings younger children are dependent on their parents to bring them to appointments, and therefore they can only access individual therapy if the parent is also engaged with the service. In the inpatient setting, this is not the case. However, the Croft is in the unique position of having both parents and children on site, allowing for close liaison with the family.

> As Philippa's therapy progressed the therapist talked to her about sharing some of the important information with her mum. Philippa was initially reluctant and so a couple of sessions focused on what Philippa thought it would be helpful for her mum to know. Philippa realised that it would be helpful for her to know quite a lot, and so a joint session was used to share the information.

For most children who have a short admission the therapeutic goals have to be carefully designed. Some children will continue to have sessions after their discharge but for some it will be more appropriate to hand over their care to a therapist in their home team. Therefore the goals of the individual sessions must allow a good collaborative formulation with the child that can be passed on to the next therapist, to agree with the child that he would like the therapy to continue and to accustom the child to a therapy model.

If there is only a short timeframe, therapy can also be contra-indicated for some difficulties. Although in some types of anxiety a few sessions might be enough to move a child on, in other types of difficulty it might not be appropriate. For example, in PTSD it might take some time for children to process their trauma, therefore starting the therapy and not being able to continue it may be counter-productive (Yule, Smith and Perrin 2004). Similarly, if there is little support for continuing an 'exposure and response prevention' intervention with a child with obsessive compulsive disorder once he has left the Croft, it might be better not to start it and to wait until the support is in place locally.

This leaves the option of working very practically with children on strategies they can use to alleviate their current distress. This is most effectively done with a collaboratively developed and agreed formulation, so children can understand why a strategy works and also so they may be able to identify new strategies by themselves (Stallard 2002).

CBT with David

David had identified that the scary things in his head were worse when he was by himself and worse when he was not doing things he enjoyed. He thought the Croft had helped because there were lots of adults to talk to and this kept the thoughts out of his head. However, when trying to make sense of his difficulties it had been worked out that when David felt scared and clung to his mum it made her cross with him and although he felt a little better that she was there, he didn't feel much better. David identified that if he was spending time by himself, playing on his computer did help and made him feel calmer. He also thought that Mum got less cross if he joined in with what the family was doing, such as watching television, rather than following her around and trying to get lots of hugs and reassurance from her. David also realised that he felt safer at his gran's house, and that he could ask Mum to let him visit Gran if things got bad. David reported that thinking about these things had been okay and that he would be keen to meet someone to talk properly about the bad things that had happened, even if he had to wait a bit. It was also agreed with David that the therapist could talk to Sarah about what he had said and a session was arranged with David and his mum to share David's worries and to help Sarah understand some of the things David felt would be helpful for her to do.

Play work

As discussed in earlier chapters, many children who come to the Croft have complex emotional issues as a result of past experiences in their lives. It is unusual for children to be able to access these underlying issues, or indeed to talk about them in a coherent way. Although children are given opportunities to talk, it is rare that they are able to put these thoughts or feelings into words. It is often through play that it is possible to provide an insight into their inner worlds. Some of the children are given this opportunity, and it is the role of the therapist to try to make sense of the material presented, and to connect with the child's life experiences (Smith 2008). In addition, relational issues may emerge through the relationship made between the play worker and child.

Usually, but not inevitably, in other settings this type of work would take place over extended periods of time (Cameron 2007). At the Croft the limited admission period has meant that these play sessions necessarily may only take place over a few weeks. The focus is therefore on assessment and the observations made in these play sessions contribute an important aspect to the overall picture obtained of the child. Importantly, it also provides an opportunity to stimulate the child's internal resources for growth and development (Shapiro 1994), and will help to indicate whether the child would benefit from longer-term play therapy.

Play sessions with David

During management meetings at the end of David's second week the team recommended that David might benefit from some play work with Jan, who ran play sessions with the children at the Croft. Staff felt that David was hard to get to know in spite of the fact that he was superficially co-operative. Given his traumatic background it was felt that it was important to get a sense of his inner world and possibly assess his suitability for longer psychotherapeutic intervention.

When Jan went to talk to David's mother, Sarah, before seeing him, Sarah was very positive about Jan working with David. Sarah expressed her frustration about the fact that David did not seem to want to talk about the physical abuse he had suffered. She saw these play sessions as a way of really finding out what was going on in David's head. She then launched at length into her own feelings of guilt about the difficult past events, becoming tearful and emotional. Jan was struck by Sarah's inability to remain focused on David's needs.

David appeared anxious as he entered the room, looking around at the toys but appearing uncertain about what to do. Jan told David that these sessions would be a bit like thinking or exploring his thoughts and feelings together. There were no right or wrong ways of doing this.

Jan noticed that he appeared to be looking at a box of football figures. She sat down on the floor and started getting the figures out of the box. David picked a figure up and said they were the wrong team. 'Oh, wrong team?' answered Jan. 'Yeah, they're losers' he said with some feeling. 'Why haven't you got West Ham footballers?' was the next question. 'West Ham supporter, are you?' David grunted an affirmative and then suddenly seemed disinterested and turned his attention to the marble run. He turned his back to her and put it together carefully and skilfully, muttering to himself during the construction. When Jan commented on how he seemed to have made an interesting route for the marbles, David ignored her. At the end of the session, Jan said: 'See you next week,' and David walked out barely looking at her.

Although Jan was pleased that David had come willingly to the first session, she was left feeling excluded and incompetent. She felt that the only emotional response she had seen had been connected with the football and was struck by his sudden disinterest and change of activity.

The next two sessions followed a similar pattern. In the third session, he became quite angry, hitting one of the footballers' heads against the floor. Jan commented: 'You're hitting the footballer really hard on the floor. Looks like you really want to hurt him.' David reacted by storming out of the room. Later in the day Jan met David in the corridor and said she was sorry that he had felt that he had had to leave but that she would be pleased to see him again next week. When thinking about the work, the themes that seemed to be emerging were: ambivalence, anger and rejection. Jan also wondered whether there were connections with his relationship with his father. On the one hand, he wanted to relate to his father through their common interest in West Ham; on the other hand, he was still confused and angry about the past abuse he had suffered from his father. Perhaps he was excluding Jan in the same way that he felt cross with his mother both for leaving his father and failing to prevent the abuse.

In their final session together, David appeared calmer. He still appeared engrossed with his football figures but became lighter and more playful on the marble run, giggling when his marble was faster than Jan's. He also made a small LEGO construction, and was more accepting of Jan's involvement. Jan said that she had enjoyed the play sessions with David and that he had been able to show her some of his strong feelings, which he had not been able to do elsewhere during his admission. She wondered whether he might like further play sessions after leaving the Croft.

Short-term music therapy at the Croft

Many of the children who come to the Croft enjoy music making and are motivated to come to music therapy sessions where there are opportunities to play instruments and improvise. As a result it is often possible to boost children's self-esteem and confidence in these sessions. For children who struggle with language, the non-verbal aspect of music making can be reassuring and gratifying. For other children music making provides an emotional outlet, perhaps giving a frustrated child an opportunity to express anger through playing the drum kit, or a sad child a chance to improvise in a quiet and sensitive way.

> During the first two weeks at the Croft it became apparent that Nick and his mother, Stacey, had an intense but difficult relationship. On the one hand, Nick appeared to be too dependent on his mother for a boy of 11 (e.g. seeking her out for hugs every two or three hours); on the other hand, he would often be aggressive and unpleasant to her, when they did spend time together. It was decided that Nick and Stacey would be offered four weekly music therapy sessions together, where the emphasis would be on allowing the two of them to enjoy making music together, to relax and have fun without feeling they needed to fulfil any particular role or show specific abilities.
>
> Nick and Stacey were both happy to come to the music room together. Nick had heard from Arthur that the drum kit was cool and Stacey said that she liked music. However, she was also slightly

self-conscious, saying that she had enjoyed playing the cornet briefly as a child, but had not been able to continue because her mother's boyfriend at the time had felt she was no good at it, and decided that it was a waste of time.

Once in the music room, Amelia explained that the purpose of the session was to enjoy playing music together. She suggested that Nick should start on the drum kit, gave Stacey a large drum and a cymbal to play, and went to the piano herself. Amelia started playing a rhythmic piece that matched the beats that Nick had initiated on the drum kit. Stacey initially looked embarrassed but then started hitting the drum herself. Amelia supported the two percussion players while slightly increasing the volume and speed of the playing. Nick experimented with different sequences of drums and Amelia matched his changing rhythm. Then Stacey played a flourish which ended on the cymbal and again Amelia echoed this phrase, but then started again with a steady pulse, to keep the improvisation going. After about five minutes the piece came to a natural end. Nick and Stacey seemed relaxed, and Amelia suggested that perhaps this time Nick would like to choose instruments for the three of them. She then suggested that they should each take it in turns to choose instruments for everyone to play.

Nick chose the electric keyboard, gave his mum a guitar and Amelia a conga drum. He seemed to want to choose proper instruments rather than tambourines or bells which he felt were 'rubbish' and babyish. On the keyboard, Nick was initially hesitant, saying he didn't know how to play. When Amelia showed him how to push buttons to get a rhythmic pattern he quickly got going and started experimenting. Stacey was trying out a chord or two on the guitar as she had been shown a few years ago. Amelia encouraged her by smiling and playing an even clear pulse on the conga. Neither Nick nor Stacey was aware of each other's playing as they were each engrossed in their own musical explorations. Eventually Amelia attempted to link up the group by improvising a song that matched both Nick's rhythm and Stacey's chords. The use of the voice surprised Nick and Stacey who both looked up and became more conscious of the other sounds being produced in the room.

After the session when Nick had returned to school Stacey and Amelia reflected on what had occurred. Stacey said she had really enjoyed playing. She said that music was something she and Nick had always liked. She then quickly returned to how difficult Nick's general behaviour was, visibly becoming anxious again as she spoke. Amelia tried to bring Stacey back to the positive session they had just had, asking her what she felt was different about this session. She said it was because Nick liked the instruments, nothing to do with her. Amelia asked whether she would mind if the session was videotaped the following week so they could look back carefully to what had happened in the session.

Two weeks later, when Stacey watched herself and Nick playing together on the video, she looked proud of Nick's keyboard playing, saying that he seemed to make up nice tunes. She asked whether she could take a copy of the video home as she wanted to show her friend. Amelia said that Nick probably got his musical sensitivity from Stacey as she had sung songs to him when he was little and they had often enjoyed listening to music together. Stacey became tearful, telling Amelia again how she had always wished she could have continued to learn the cornet when she was little. She was also visibly moved that she was being told that there was an aspect of her mothering that was successful.

In their last session together, Amelia made sure they spent some time on wind instruments, giving Stacey the recorder, Nick two reed horns and improvising on the clarinet herself. At times they all played together, at others they took it in turns, echoing and imitating each other's phrases. At one point Nick missed a note and a really funny noise was produced...this made all three of them laugh and they had to stop playing. Over the weeks Nick had become more and more confident, sometimes learning short tunes on the keyboard which he then played to other children at the Croft. He had generally become more aware of what both his mum and Amelia were doing while he was playing. He was warm and caring towards his mother, always trying to choose instruments for her that she would like.

Stacey was always positive about the sessions but struggled not to be overwhelmed by her difficulties generally. She gradually realised that she could enjoy music again without always feeling regretful about the past and, most importantly, she began to acknowledge that she had played a part in helping Nick to be a sensitive musician and could be proud of this.

Summary

There are many different types of assessments on offer for children who come to the Croft. With such a variety on offer within a short timeframe it is important not to overwhelm the child, and to balance the individual assessments with the group- or family-based assessments described in other chapters. However, an advantage of multi-modal intensive assessment is that each assessment can quickly build on previous ones, based on hypotheses derived at the start of the admission, and developed each week in team meetings and supervision. Inconsistencies can easily be explored and gaps can be filled. The flexibility of the approach allows for a coherent, integrated formulation to develop over time. To make this approach work, frequent and clear communication within the team and constant development of the hypotheses and formulation are needed. With this a useful formulation that takes into account the important aspects of the child's experience and characteristics can be developed, that in turn leads to useful discussions with the child and family about how to help them reach their goals.

Chapter 9

Understanding the Family

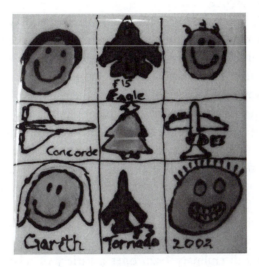

The important things in Gareth's life were
his family, planes and Christmas

Introduction

Previous chapters have focused on assessment and treatment for the individual child. This chapter considers the family as the patient and how the strengths and difficulties of the family unit are assessed, and describes therapy directed at the family group.

As mentioned previously, the Croft is at present the only child and family psychiatric inpatient service in the UK to routinely admit children and family members as inpatients. The reasons for this include a belief that children can only be assessed holistically if their family relationships are also assessed. Also, it is clear from decades of research that there can be a reciprocal relationship between problems in the child and problems in the family, particularly for children with the most complex needs (Hyland 1990). There is a growing body of evidence that documents the efficacy of family therapy as an integral part of a psychiatric treatment plan (for a review see McFarlane *et al.* 2003), resulting in improved patient recovery, reduced relapse rates, improved family wellbeing and reduced costs for care. This suggests that family-based interventions benefit both service providers and patients and their families. As a result, working with families is integral to the unit's practice.

In this chapter the 'why, how and what' regarding the practice of family therapy within the unit programme is explored. This work creates a vital forum for each family to consider their own situation and to explore both the family history and the family future.

Being away from home with none of the usual work or domestic tasks, sharing a communal space with other families and professionals, whilst being continually observed, generates considerable stress, especially in the early weeks. Many parents describe the pressure cooker or fish bowl effect of becoming resident in the Croft.

However, the experience, which offers a variety of contexts for children and parents to relate to each other, also provides them with a safe environment in which they can practise alternative ways of interacting.

The multi-disciplinary team offer a variety of relationships and experiences for children and parents, but the nursing team in particular create the climate for an integrated approach as described in Chapters 3 and 4. The formal family therapy session offers the opportunity to consider all these experiences and place them in the context of the life of the family. The family therapists have a particular role to keep in mind the wider system: the family at home, the referring agency and other professionals involved with the family referrer (Palazzoli *et al.* 1980b).

Principles of family therapy that inform the practice at the Croft

A number of beliefs underpin the position taken in family therapy at the unit (Hesketh and Olney 2004).

> *People do their best*: this is central to most family therapy practice and is essential in maintaining the neutrality required to see each part of the system as benignly intended (Palazzoli *et al.* 1980a). An example of how this principle might create new ways of

thinking would be to consider abusive behaviour. Whilst on the surface abuse towards children by parents would be universally decried, if one starts from the premise that the parents are trying to do their best, their abusive behaviour could be understood to be an attempt to protect their children or to show love in a way that might reflect the parents' own experience of being parented.

'No one truth and no one model': This is a natural consequence of neutrality as there are many ways of understanding any single event or relationship. This reflects the influence of post-modernism on family therapy, which as a result remains open to multiple truths. Each part of the system, including family members, the unit team, other professionals and the wider society, may have different truths and different ways of understanding any given event.

Similarly, the family therapists remain open to a range of theoretical models within both the family therapy field and those embraced by other disciplines. For example, within a child mental health inpatient unit, the whole spectrum of interventions (medical, behavioural, systemic, psychodynamic, psycho-educational, social and legal) is embraced. Clearly, family therapy privileges the systemic understandings and respects all the models within its own discipline. Some schools of family therapy such as solution-focused therapy (de Shazer 1988; George, Iveson and Ratner 1990) do not place great weight on understanding 'why' people behave the way they do, but within a multi-disciplinary assessment and treatment programme an understanding of the origins and meanings of presenting behaviours is necessary as part of creating a cohesive, meaningful care plan for a child and her family which will inform their ongoing relationship with agencies.

Respecting difference: maintaining openness to models and respecting neutrality leads to embracing differences between types of people, both family and professionals. This means giving a voice to children, parents, stepparents, grandparents and other relatives and also listening to the views of all members of the unit team regardless of their position in the professional hierarchy. Great emphasis is placed on inclusion of the fathers and stepfathers as they are usually the parent least likely to be resident on the unit. Grandparents are regularly included in outpatient therapy. Siblings also have much to say as they have frequently had to tolerate huge disruption in their daily lives and to accept that the 'problem' child absorbs so much of their parents' time. This leads to the index child often being seen as the favourite or alternatively as responsible for all the problems in the family.

Respecting difference also requires the therapists to be open about their own prejudices, something that is explored within the family therapy team and within the wider staff team through group supervision and the externally facilitated staff support meeting.

Transference: this is a concept that has come from classical psychoanalysis and is used to describe the intense emotions that families project on to the therapists that have their origin in important emotional experiences and relationships elsewhere in their lives. Transference from families and patients is mirrored by *counter-transference*, the process whereby therapists bring feelings from their own experiences into the therapy session. Being aware of these processes helps the therapists to understand and manage the often highly emotive differences and prejudices that emerge during therapeutic sessions.

Some families create particularly intense emotional responses in the staff team which can often be usefully understood in terms of the feelings projected into the staff by members of the family. For example, a parent may evoke feelings of frustration amongst certain staff members and this can lead to a wish to 'rescue' the child from that parent. At the same time other members of the team can feel very sympathetic to the parents and be very aware of their emotional vulnerability; these team members may want to protect the parents from criticism or confrontation. This 'splitting' of responses is not unusual and is a warning to the staff team to find time to reflect on the feelings and prejudices that are created by this parent. If the position of rescuing the child is maintained, it is likely that the parent will be undermined and punished, and if the protective position is privileged, then the risk of harm to the child may not be addressed.

Hope versus hopelessness: this is a very common theme for many families. Many parents come to the unit after many years of confusion and uncertainty due to the complexity of their child's difficulties. Often they have seen many professionals without significant progress. In this situation both parents and therapists may be torn between hope and hopelessness. Whilst the therapists maintain a stance of tentative curiosity, privileging the positives, it is important to be aware of the dangers of being unrealistic and overly hopeful. This tension is particularly prominent when working with families who have been referred for parenting capacity assessments from a court or the child protection agencies. It is tempting to be drawn into the position of 'the rule of optimism' that was described by Louis Blom-Cooper in the Beckford Child Protection Inquiry, where he highlighted that maintaining hope for change could mask the risks to children (Blom-Cooper 1985). Family therapy sessions can provide a forum for this tension to be voiced and the gap between what is hoped for and what is to be explored can be defined.

What prevents competence: this is a question that is continually raised when families are struggling to manage ordinary day-to-day tasks or to prevent extraordinary events happening in their families. Most parents have a range of skills to be competent and effective in their parenting task so it is useful to ask what constrains this. For example, a parent may have been observed on the unit being loving and emotionally warm to a child from another resident family, but being unable to show the same level of emotional warmth to her own child. Usually when this kind of discrepancy is discussed, connections with the parent's own experiences of childhood are discovered. For example, parents who see intimacy as sexualised (from their own experience of sexual abuse) may be anxious about intimacy with their own children and find ways to avoid it.

Solutions versus dilemmas: traditional approaches to problem-solving expect to find solutions. Systemic therapy is underpinned by a belief that there are both positive and negative aspects to changes in behaviour as there are also positive and negative aspects to a 'no change' position, that is, staying as you are. As

Barry Mason (1993) states: solutions are a myth because they are only dilemmas that are less worrying than the previous dilemma. He goes on to argue for the importance of creating a context of 'safe uncertainty', an idea that is similar to the psychodynamic concept of 'containment', something that the Croft team tries to create both for the families and for other professionals. For example, it is acknowledged that both parents and children may wish to express a range of feelings about their predicament. Some of these may be focused on themselves, the Croft team or the wider professional system.

The attempted solution becomes the problem: this is a common formulation in systemic therapy. For example, a child may resolve the problem of a parent's loneliness by staying at home but this leads to school refusal and means the child missing out on school and friends. Similarly, an over-helpful professional system may undermine parental confidence.

How family therapy is conducted

Each family has a family therapy session at least weekly and there are often different combinations of family members at different stages of therapy. The therapy sessions are led by the unit family therapist, a family therapy trained member of staff or sometimes family therapy trainees under close supervision. Therapy sessions often start with the resident parent or parents. In the first meeting parents are asked about their hopes for their admission and their greatest worries for their child, and their professional involvements prior to admission are tracked.

The earlier sessions usually focus on gaining a full picture of the family by drawing a genogram or family tree. These sessions are also an opportunity for the parents to talk about their experiences and worries without the child/children being present. Whenever possible, the family therapy team use the reflecting team method (Andersen 1987). This involves the use of one or more clinicians to act as observers of the conversation between the therapist and the family. This observation can take place within the therapy room or with the observers sitting behind a one-way screen. Then at points within the session the reflecting team will have a conversation in front of the therapist and the family about the session they have been observing, offering tentative and enquiring thoughts on the conversation between family and therapist. The reflecting team then leave the therapy room, and the therapist and the family have the opportunity to pick up any themes that the reflecting team have raised. Using the reflecting team supports the therapist, as additional eyes and ears can note interactions between family members that the therapist in the room might miss. They also offer additional thinking space to cope with what are often complex conversations with multiple themes and views.

Parents have the right to refuse the use of the reflecting team but it is extremely rare for them to do so, and most appear interested in and pleased with the comments offered.

As suggested above, team membership is not fixed and whenever possible the key workers and other clinicians are part of the reflecting team. This helps to connect the family therapy sessions with the work of the wider team. It also has a benefit to the team of flattening the professional hierarchy and ensuring that a multi-disciplinary perspective can be taken. In the pre- and post-session team discussions, team members can comment on the progress of the family in other parts of the programme so the family therapy can incorporate feedback from the wider staff team. In the post-session discussion information arising from the family therapy session can be fed back to the wider team and incorporated into subsequent assessments or interventions. Being in the reflecting team can pose a dilemma for staff of shifting the context of their relationship with families. This is particularly pertinent for nurses and care assistants who provide the majority of the direct care to children as one minute they might be offering comments in the formal setting of the reflecting team and shortly afterwards be involved in managing an outburst in the same child. It is notable that the model of care at the unit requires all staff to be skilled at working systemically with parents and children so even relatively unqualified staff, over time, become comfortable in the reflecting team and use the model with ease.

What happens in family therapy at the Croft?

The core element of a family therapy session is a conversation conducted with the principles described above, of neutrality and respectful curiosity. Within that conversation various activities may be used to stimulate the conversation and to explore different aspects of family functioning.

Genogram

As mentioned above, the first meeting usually involves the adults, and a family tree is constructed on a large whiteboard in the therapy room. As this is gradually evolving, the therapist asks about the quality of the relationships between family members and how each important family member feels about the admission and what their hopes and fears might be.

This allows the family therapy team to be aware of both the nature of the concerns about the child and who is most concerned in the family.

For many parents this is the first time they have seen their family represented by symbols on a large whiteboard. Patterns may be readily visible across extended families. For example, relationships that have been violent and abusive or where there have been physical or emotional health concerns are clearly annotated. A frequent comment from parents is: 'Doesn't it look a mess?', and many parents find this review of their family tree to be an emotionally charged conversation. The genogram has the added effect of placing the identified child in the context of family relationships, which widens the focus. During this initial activity parents often start to consider how their child's difficulties or their own parenting style connect with events that have occurred in previous generations.

Life cycle transitions

Referrals into child mental health services often occur when a crisis has arisen as a child or family are negotiating a life cycle transition. These transitions can occur when people leave or join the family group, such as when a child is born or when someone leaves home, divorces or dies. There are also many other situations that cause family members to renegotiate their relationship pattern, such as unemployment or illness. Often, families in crisis will have to negotiate several life cycle stages during a short time period that overstretches the system's ability to reorganise itself (Carter and McGoldrick 1999).

Sometimes a problem can emerge for a child that mirrors an event in the parent's life. For example, if the parent was placed in care at the age of ten because of severe family difficulties then a crisis can arise when her own child is approaching that age. In this situation a useful question can be 'What was your life like when you were the same age as your child?' This question can trigger a discussion about connections across three generations and encourages reflection about patterns of intimacy, control and beliefs in the parent's family of origin that may be unconsciously influencing the beliefs and attributions in the current generation.

Power and authority

The use of power and authority is an important theme for most families; for those families using children's inpatient services, clarity around who can exercise authority and who holds power within the family has often become lost. Salvador Minuchin (1974) developed structural models of family therapy in the 1970s in which he described how families are organised into hierarchies that are separated by boundaries. The quality of these boundaries determines the way intimacy, power and rules are organised. Minuchin's model emphasises that parents should be in charge, and he represented this figuratively as parents being above the boundary line and children being below. Many families admitted into the Croft experience a reversal of this pattern, with the children above the line and parents below. In an alternative situation, very concerned grandparents may have taken charge, which has the unintended, but unhelpful, effect of undermining parental authority. The simple exercise of drawing a horizontal line on the whiteboard and asking family members to indicate who they feel is above the line and who is below can create a powerful visual statement about who is in charge in the family.

An attractive element of the structural model is its simplicity. Having clear family roles and responsibilities is a concept that is easily understood by both adults and children and it is particularly pertinent when working with families with pre-adolescent children. Often children who portray themselves as being above the line in their family will also talk about how uncomfortable they feel in this position and how much they want the adults to take charge.

The genogram, together with the line exercise, explores power relations within the family and combines structural and trans-generational approaches to family therapy. The aim is to help families see their problems as embedded within a wider system and also to help them to see how patterns unfold over time. This is often the first step in uncovering the issues that are preventing parents from exercising their full competence. For example, parents who experienced serious physical abuse from their own parents may be desperate not to repeat this behaviour with their own children and thus may feel that any type of control or discipline is abusive. Such parents frequently step back from setting firm boundaries for fear of feeling abusive. The child may then experience a sense that it doesn't matter what she does, and her behaviour escalates in an attempt to elicit an appropriate parental response. The child and the parent may then become locked in an unhappy pattern of increasing aggression from the child and increasing withdrawal and victimisation by the parents. This can reach a point where parents experience their own child as causing the same fear that they experienced during their own childhood abuse.

Sometimes such conversations about trauma experienced in childhood by the parent allow the therapists to enquire about intense and often disturbing feelings that are evoked. These post-traumatic stress responses may also constrain parents from exercising their parental skills. Sometimes parents have been unable to discuss their own childhood trauma before and they have needed the wrap-around care of an inpatient admission to feel contained and safe enough to start to explore such sensitive issues. This places the family therapy team in a therapeutic dilemma, as clearly it is important to explore this part of the family history, but it is equally important to ensure that parents will have access to ongoing therapeutic support after their discharge.

Challenging violence

Some parents who come into the Croft experience considerable violence from their children. They often believe that the aggression stems from an inherent disorder in the child's brain functioning and they hope that professionals might be able to alter the child in some way to reduce this behaviour. This issue can be more complex if the child is felt to have a mental health diagnosis but the structural model would still suggest that the parent's role is to hold the boundaries firm.

The structural model of family therapy challenges the belief that the child has no control over her body due to having a mental health diagnosis. We challenge this directly, using ideas from Alan Jenkins (1990) and Minuchin (1974; Minuchin and Fishman 1981) to inform our practice. Jenkins wrote about the concept of 'entitlement', which is discussed with the parents to explore possible explanations about where the children learnt their entitlement to control others by violence. This approach also reflects the assumption contained in the structural model of family therapy premised on the belief that children are in charge of their own bodies, although we recognise that self-control is likely to be more difficult for a child who experiences major distress.

Minuchin (Minuchin and Fishman 1981) would invite such children to punch his hand during a family session and then talk to the child about how her brain had to listen to his instruction and then send a message to the muscles in her hands and then aim to deliver the punch which had then to be accurately directed towards Minuchin's hand. This exercise highlighted to both children and parents that hitting is not a spontaneous event out of the child's conscious control but a complex movement that has to be planned and carefully executed to be effective.

When this technique is used within family sessions at the Croft most children are initially confused as they will not have experienced a professional inviting a punch before. Most parents find the exercise helpful and it can stimulate a very valuable discussion about taking responsibility for one's own actions. Other families may find the exercise an uncomfortable one because if their child's aggression can be controlled, this might mean that they and their child could find a solution by acting differently rather than waiting for a solution from outside the family.

Accommodation

Most children coming to child mental health units show extreme behaviours, but if these behaviours are tracked backwards, it is often discovered that they started with a modest eccentricity or mildly antisocial behaviour. For example, a child who is admitted with severely obsessional behaviour may have originally shown mild pickiness about food or a tendency to dislike getting her hands messy.

These mild idiosyncrasies may be accepted and tolerated by parents for a variety of justifiable reasons; maybe because they love their child and do not want to make her feel embarrassed or because they have similar traits and do not think they are a problem. In this situation parents often believe that the symptom will worsen if attention is drawn to it or that it is a passing phase.

Within weeks all family members can learn to accept one member's 'odd' behaviour so that it becomes considered 'normal'. If the symptom does progress it becomes increasingly eccentric until it becomes a debilitating concern. For families who wish to avoid conflict, their care, love and wish to accept their child, whatever the problem, may then lead to a denial of the severity of the problem. This may cause parents to see professional concern as worsening their child's problem. This is an example of the systemic principle that the attempted solution (accommodating the problem behaviour) may become the problem (Watzlawick, Weakland and Fisch 1974). In this situation it is vital to form a collaborative approach between parents and professionals, and family therapy can support this by acknowledging the parents' care of their child whilst supporting them to challenge the dysfunctional symptom. An exploration of the roots of the family's discomfort with managing conflict can also help to free up the situation.

Sculpting

This technique was developed in the USA in the 1960s by Duhl and his colleagues (Duhl, Kantor and Duhl 1973). It is active and uses space rather than words to highlight relationship patterns. Each member of the family is asked in turn to sculpt the family members, that is, to place them in the room in a way that represents how they get on together, and this demonstrates closeness versus distance and the hierarchy in the family. All the family members are then invited to describe how they feel in the position that they have been placed in. Each family member can have their turn to sculpt the family both as it is and also how they would like it to be if they had a magic wand.

For example, a mother may place the index child standing on the coffee table whilst her partner and other children sit on the floor. This sculpt would vividly illustrate that the child is in charge. Another sculpt could reveal visually that one parent or grandparent is very close and involved with the child at the expense of the other parent's involvement with that child. In the sculpt it can often be seen that this physical closeness prevents the more distant parent from even being able to see the child. It also demonstrates that for any better contact to be made one parent needs to step back in order to allow the other parent to step forward and have greater access to the child.

A less physically demanding version of sculpting uses objects, such as LEGO bricks, to represent family members – children can find this a more approachable exercise as they are used to handling LEGO and are skilled at using different pieces of LEGO for different building tasks. Children and adults can be asked to place different LEGO pieces on a coffee table to represent family relationships.

This use of physical movement or objects to represent relationships can be particularly helpful with families who find talking about relationships difficult. It can also be used to track changes in relationship patterns by repeating the exercise as the admission and therapy progress.

Projective identification

Borrowing from psychodynamic theory, the concept of projective identification is connected to transference and has been explored in the systemic literature by Flaskas (1996). This concept refers to the idea that a negative emotion that cannot be acknowledged becomes transmitted to another person and expressed by that person.

Some children seem to show no pattern to their behaviour and can, for example, be constantly angry or randomly violent. In talking to their parents about their own lives, it may emerge that one of them carries strong feelings of anger or aggression that they cannot express and have put a great deal of energy into concealing. Often the parent complains of depression rather than any outwardly directed negative emotion. The child's violence can then be thought of as an expression of intense loyalty to her parent as she acts out the feelings that emanate from that parent. In other words, the child is expressing the emotion that the parent cannot.

In this situation conversations in family therapy (and elsewhere during the admission) can help adults to acknowledge their own feelings. If the adults can learn to express their own emotions then it is hoped that the need for the child to show them on their behalf will lessen.

Circular questioning

Family therapy has evolved a vast array of questioning techniques designed to encourage family members to be self-reflective. The Milan team (Palazzoli *et al.* 1980a) developed this area in the 1970s and contributed an approach known as circular questioning to the field. This approach has been further developed by other therapists, notably Karl Tomm (1987) and Peggy Penn (1982). Circular questioning is designed to draw out connections between emotions and behaviour within family relationships and to see these connections as circular rather than linear. So, for example, rather than asking why a mother is depressed (a linear question), the therapist might ask who in the family is most affected by the mother's depression (a circular question). This approach aims to open up new ways of thinking for the family, and for the family to think of themselves as all involved in an interconnected system.

Therapeutic letter writing

White and Epston (1989) developed the use of therapeutic letters. After each meeting the family therapist writes a letter to the parents summarising the conversation. The aim is to provide the family with an opportunity to reflect further on the session, to share the themes of the session with other team members working with the family and also to create an ongoing account of the family's path through therapy. Reflecting the wish to promote openness, families know that the therapists will not write anything in a report about them that has not been included in the post-session letters. They are also aware that the letter records the therapist's impression of the session and they may have different recollections. Different views may well stimulate further useful discussion in the next session.

An additional benefit of therapeutic letter writing is that the therapist can include thoughts and themes that emerge in the therapy team's post-session discussion, and again these additional ideas may be a useful starting point for the next therapy session. Some writers expound the virtues of therapeutic letters (Fox 2003), suggesting they multiply the impact of the face-to-face therapy. Within the families using the service, feedback has been mixed. Some parents have found them very useful and have shown the letters to family members who were not in the session leading to a continuation of the therapeutic conversation with the wider family. Other parents do not read the letters and some parents worry that each letter may be seen as the final view of their family situation even though it is stressed that parents are able to amend or challenge what is written.

Therapeutic letters reflect the dilemma, experienced in many parts of the programme, of balancing the aim to stimulate positive change with an assessment of the capacity of parents to meet their children's needs. Whilst the letters attempt to be an accurate summary of the content and process of the dilemmas presented in each session, a deliberate effort is made to privilege the themes of hope and change. If these letters then, at a later date, form part of evidence in legal or child protection processes, they may not fully reflect the concerns of the therapeutic team. This is the tension of working therapeutically in a setting where the context shifts, and therapists must be mindful of being clear about their role, as outlined by Cecchin (1987) and Lang and Little (1990), and be aware of which 'hat' they are wearing at any given time.

Challenges of family therapy in an intensive residential setting

The limited timeframe of admissions means the family therapists have to work quickly and at a level of intensity that would be inappropriate in outpatient settings. For example, the genogram is usually an intense and emotional experience where parents may have a sense of being laid bare in the first session. In outpatient work families might only undertake this after one or two orientation sessions. However, since parents in the unit are able to seek support from staff directly after a session, the therapeutic pace can be faster.

Earlier the ethical dilemmas of the limited length of stay, especially when family members are exploring deeply troubling events which influence their parenting, were referred to. Many parents report that family therapy is the most challenging aspect of the admission but they also often develop a sense of trust in the unit's family therapy team, and having shared very sensitive discussions about their family life, they are understandably reluctant to restart these conversations and relationships with therapists in their local areas. In addition families are often just starting to explore important areas in therapy as the admission finishes, and the transition from intensive inpatient care to being back in the community can create further tensions. For all these reasons, the family therapy team have developed a package of follow-up therapy sessions, every three to four weeks, for up to six months after the family's discharge. This is discussed with the referring team in the discharge meeting and offered to families where ongoing family therapy is felt to be an important part of their care plan. Wherever possible, this post-admission package includes handover sessions with the local team so that the therapeutic work can be dovetailed into any local support that is in place.

This follow-up work seems most effective when families have already used the therapy sessions to make significant changes during their residential stay but want more time and support to consolidate these changes. This also fits with the outcome research of Green *et al.* (2007) that suggests that longer periods of intervention are associated with more effective long-term change in families.

Case example

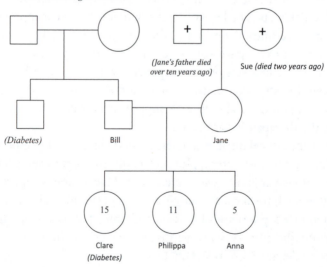

Family tree: Jane (mum), Bill (dad), Clare (sister), Philippa, Anna (sister) and Sue (maternal grandmother)

Retired and living in France

(Jane's father died over ten years ago)   Sue *(died two years ago)*

(Diabetes)   Bill   Jane

15   11   5

Clare   Philippa   Anna
(Diabetes)

Figure 9.1 Genogram of Philippa's family

Philippa was admitted to the Croft because of rapid weight loss that appeared to be triggered by the sudden death of her maternal grandmother. Philippa had always been a picky eater from her toddler years and she became vegetarian when she was nine years old. This meant that, for the last two years, her mother, Jane, had cooked separate meals for her. Both parents reluctantly accepted Philippa's choice to be vegetarian but had always worried that she might not be having a balanced diet. Bill was worried that this was an extra burden on his wife as she did the bulk of the day-to-day parenting, since his job kept him away from home for one to two weeks each month.

Whenever possible, Bill had visited his eldest daughter, Clare, in hospital during her frequent admissions due to her severe diabetes. Although Clare's illness had been successfully managed she was likely to continue to need frequent medical check-ups and she was at risk of further medical problems in adulthood. Philippa had always been anxious about her older sister, particularly when she had needed to be hospitalised.

In the initial family therapy session their genogram was drawn on the whiteboard. Philippa's family were experiencing several life cycle transitions. Philippa was about to move into secondary school whilst Clare was starting to talk about leaving home to go to college and their youngest daughter, Anna, had started primary school. Recently Jane's beloved mother Sue had died unexpectedly. Sue had been a huge support to Jane and had developed a particularly close relationship with Philippa as she had cared for her whenever Clare was in hospital. This was seen as a helpful balance to the reduced time that Jane could devote to Philippa. Bill's parents were both healthy but had retired to France so had infrequent contact with the family.

It became clear that Sue had been a central figure in the family. Her involvement with the family had intensified after the birth of Philippa so that Jane and Bill could continue to focus on Clare's health. Clare had many admissions to hospital as a younger child. Meanwhile, as Bill's career progressed he was spending more time out of the country and Sue's role became even more significant. All the family agreed that Philippa ate best when she was staying with Sue, and she often talked about her grandmother's good cooking.

As the sessions proceeded it became clear that there was a lack of clarity about power and authority in the family. This prompted a session involving a family sculpt. The family members were invited to place each other in the room in a way that reflected how they perceived family relationships to be. Sue's role was represented by one of the reflecting team.

Clare was the first to have a try. Using small dolls, she placed her mum and grandmother standing in the middle of the room, with her sisters, her dad and herself kneeling on the floor next to them. She placed Bill's hands on the shoulders of both his elder daughters but with his face looking away from the family. Everyone agreed this arrangement made sense although all three adults said they felt uncomfortable in their positions. Philippa then wanted to change the layout and she placed Clare in the centre with the other five family members in a circle around her. Once again the family members all said how this arrangement also made sense but Clare said being surrounded by her family made her feel selfish and claustrophobic.

Each family member was invited to comment on their feelings about these two sculpts and Jane immediately expressed her concern that her husband was not alongside her in the first sculpt. Bill picked up on her comment and said that he thought it was an accurate reflection of the importance and power of Sue in their family. He talked about how grateful he had been for her support but that it had also made him feel somewhat on the periphery of the family. He said that he had always felt too guilty to voice this feeling. Jane acknowledged that Bill had always felt devastated and guilty about Clare's illness and that she thought he had partially withdrawn from the family and dedicated himself to his job as his way of coping.

The first sculpt had highlighted the vital role of Sue and all the family agreed that she had felt like the main support to Jane. This meant that Sue had become the co-parent and shared most of the parenting authority. Bill acknowledged that the more central Sue had become the more he tended to withdraw. He didn't like to express his anger because he recognised the continual strain on Jane.

Jane described her intense sadness at the loss of her mother and her fear that she wouldn't manage to keep the family going without her. Jane, like her husband, was reluctant to express any anger, anger at Bill, anger about the burden of life with a sick child, or anger about the additional burden of Philippa's illness.

The second sculpt aroused strong responses in Clare as Philippa, for the first time, was able to say how she had often felt like the 'Cinderella' in the family but hated herself for having those thoughts. Clare said she had always felt guilty about the burden of her illness but also acknowledged that it was sometimes a comfort to know that she was always going to be the focus of love and attention regardless of how she behaved.

Bill said that he thought Philippa was greatly missing her grandmother and Philippa quietly agreed by nodding her head. She then said that nothing tasted any good since her grandmother had died.

The family were then asked to re-arrange the sculpt in their ideal way. Dad immediately placed himself where Sue had been. Jane looked delighted and the girls looked relieved and they arranged themselves on either side of their parents.

This simple exercise powerfully demonstrates relationship patterns that had emerged over the years as this family struggled to find ways to cope. It seemed that Philippa's sudden weight loss flagged up the crisis as this family had to reconfigure its pattern of relating. There followed, in later sessions, lengthy explorations of the loss of Sue and the shift in Bill and Jane's relationship. For the first time, they could also speak about the impact of Clare's illness on them as parents and as a couple. They agreed strategies to support one another to ensure Philippa ate a healthier diet.

In one session both girls talked about the impact of Clare's diabetes; Philippa managed to talk about her mixture of guilt that her sister had to suffer whilst also acknowledging her anger at the impact on family life and her relationship with her parents. Clare, meanwhile, was able to describe her own anger at her illness which had dominated her childhood whilst at the same time feeling furious at Philippa for her 'self-inflicted' illness that was controlling family life. Both Clare and Philippa expressed concern that the needs of Anna, as a five-year-old, were sometimes overlooked because of their respective needs.

The themes discussed in the sessions were shared with Philippa's key workers. Family meals were arranged and the nurses devised ways to actively support both Jane and Bill in their new strategy to 'speak with one voice' in their resolve to not let Philippa take charge of her eating. Jane and Bill were reclaiming their shared authority over their daughter.

Summary

The assessment and treatment of any child with complex mental health problems should always include the family. This chapter has focused on the role of family therapy within a child and family mental health unit in terms of both assessing and treating the family system. Basic assumptions that the family are doing their best and maintaining a neutral and respectful standpoint underpin family therapy and the team's outlook.

Admitting families to the inpatient unit creates an opportunity for intensive therapy. The wrap-around nature of the care team and the many opportunities for reflection give families an opportunity to practise new ways of relating. The family therapy sessions support this process and ensure that members of the family who are not admitted are also involved in the therapeutic process. The systemic model of thinking and the focus on clear roles and boundaries in the family permeates the whole programme but is made very explicit in the family sessions.

Chapter 10

Creating a New Story

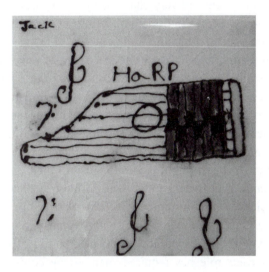

Jack wanted to be remembered by the harp

Mixed feelings

The beginnings and ends of all human undertakings are untidy.

John Galsworthy

The good news for families, even those involved in very intensive work with professionals, is that eventually that involvement comes to an end. For some families this is a great relief, especially if they have been working with many different professionals from many agencies. Often ordinary life has been overtaken by appointments and visits and telephone calls. Families may have been exposed to frequent questioning and sometimes critical appraisal of the way they are conducting their family life.

However, despite the turmoil that professional involvement can cause, sometimes the approach of the end of contact can evoke mixed feelings. Parents may feel anxious, if practical or emotional support is to reduce or stop – they might have formed close and confiding relationships with workers to the point that the worker may have a more intimate knowledge of their life and emotions than close family members. Naturally, ending such a relationship will cause a sense of loss. Parents may also be left managing situations and behaviours with their children that are still very challenging in themselves, and along with this comes the realisation that despite everyone's best efforts there will be ongoing difficulties to live with.

Children, depending on their age and stage of development, can also have a strong emotional response to moving out of treatment or support. They may also have formed positive attachments to workers, particularly if there has been a series of individual sessions as part of their treatment plan. They may also mirror their parents' worries or fear that everything will return to the way it was when the family were in the crisis that brought professionals into their lives originally.

At the same time professionals will also be dealing with their own ambivalence at ending contact – hope that things will go well for a family mixed with anxieties that they may not. Sometimes professionals will be relieved at the end of a period of involvement, especially if their role has required them to be confrontational or challenging. In other situations workers can become very warmly attached to the families they work with and so will also find endings times of loss.

All of these scenarios are very familiar to an inpatient team. After weeks of getting to know a family and working alongside them, leaving is usually an emotional time. Sometimes behaviours may reappear that had resolved previously, or parents may find their confidence is less strong – given these factors the team must work together to ensure that families can use this phase, often characterised by uncertainty and ambivalence, to move back into their community and ordinary life with the best chance of holding onto, and building on, the progress that they have made.

> Philippa is in her last week at the unit – she has been gradually spending more and more time at home and has had some time in her own school in the last couple of weeks. Philippa's parents have established a regular routine at home for meals. This has gone well and she has reached her healthy weight range.

Philippa's mum mentions to their key worker that Philippa has been talking at home about how much she hates how her body looks, particularly her thighs. Jane is wondering if Philippa is ready to be discharged or if she needs more time on the unit to feel happier about her body.

The team discuss this and feel that it is understandable that Philippa will continue to have thoughts she will struggle with. It is also understandable that her mum may be feeling anxious about coping once Philippa has been discharged. The key worker arranges to meet with Jane and Philippa to remind them how much progress they have made, to go over the care plan that will be in place after they leave and emphasise there will be ongoing telephone support and that they will be coming back for some further family therapy sessions.

A key component of the work with families is the creation of a new or amended vision of themselves and the challenges they are facing. Families arrive feeling stressed and emotionally distraught. Often they feel they have no power to change the situation they are in and they feel worn down and hopeless. In addition they often feel frustrated by the professional system, frustrated by a lack of clarity about their child's difficulties or a lack of services or interventions to support them. So the team works together to give parents, children and, families a chance to experience successes, to re-focus on strengths and feel empowered to manage the difficulties they live with.

The team start thinking about the end of an intervention at the outset. It is essential to keep a focus on the therapeutic aims, to create realistic goals as well as to acknowledge what cannot be changed. A practical arrangement that reinforces this focus is to set a date for a network meeting to be held during the last week of a family's stay. This is booked as the family start working with the service and this helps the team to keep in mind the other professionals working with the family and to be mindful of the important role that they have and that they are the team that will provide ongoing care. This network meeting will involve the family, the child's school, family doctor, paediatric and/or mental health specialists, social care worker and anyone else that the family want to be involved. The meeting is called a discharge meeting but the team see it as the beginning of a new phase of work, as the family return to their home and re-engage with community services.

The discharge meeting

For most parents, this meeting, which brings together many professionals, and marks the end of their stay and re-engagement with their local services, is an anxiety-provoking event. They and their children are under the spotlight and they will be meeting professionals again that they last met when they were in crisis.

An important part of this meeting is the preparation – all the team members who are submitting reports to this meeting discuss them with the parents during the days running up to the meeting. This gives parents the opportunity to ask questions, to challenge opinions and to ensure that their views are included in the feedback and that they are not faced with new pieces of information in a large and, potentially, intimidating meeting. Parents are encouraged to add their own comments to the reports so that they feel ownership of the information rather than passive recipients. They also have their own space in the meeting to give their report and their feedback about their treatment, emphasising their prominence in the process.

The voice of the child

Meetings with large groups of adults are not usually very child-friendly and yet it is of course vital that the child's views and wishes are heard and play a key role in shaping the ongoing plan for his care and support. Ensuring that the voice of the child is heard is challenging, and many agencies have put a great deal of work into finding the best way to help children speak up for themselves when decisions are being made about their treatment, support and care.

Built into the inpatient programme are opportunities for children to meet with staff members individually, and key workers use these sessions to find out how the children see their situation and how they want it to be different – this can be done through talking sessions, play sessions, music sessions or informal interactions such as being pushed on a swing or making a LEGO model.

More recently the organisation have commissioned an advocacy organisation to provide a service to children at the unit.

Advocacy with children with complex difficulties

The role of advocacy is to provide a neutral adult who will listen to a child, young person or vulnerable adult without an agenda of her own, to hear the child's views and represent these to others when the person in question cannot do this directly. Advocates may also help their clients to understand issues that are pertinent to their lives.

Part of the role of the advocate for children in hospital is to ensure that the care that they receive is safe and appropriate.

Advocacy has its roots in the human rights movement that emerged during the twentieth century and the importance of advocacy has been highlighted during investigations of institutional abuse of children and vulnerable adults. Serious case reviews addressing these scandals have identified that one of the risk factors for abuse is a closed system, that is, situations where outside visitors are unwelcome and the children and young people have few or no opportunities to speak to adults outside the institution.

Over time advocacy services have expanded to seek the views of children and vulnerable adults in many situations where they are marginalised and important decisions are being made about their lives without enough consideration being taken of their viewpoint.

In an inpatient setting with an average stay of six weeks the challenge for advocates is considerable – they have to form a relationship with a child over a relatively short time period, and many of the children find questions about what they think or feel particularly difficult to answer because of their developmental and/or emotional difficulties. It has become clear that it is vital for advocates to spend time with the children in fun and relaxed situations – usually playing games or taking part in a craft session – before they can usefully attempt to talk to them about their wishes and feelings. The advocate at the Croft uses child-friendly worksheets to ask the children about their views of the service, both positive and negative, and also about what changes they would like to see in their lives after they leave.

Having an advocate coming onto the unit has been especially helpful to the team when they have become over-focused on the parents' needs or views and it has ensured that the team also hears the children's views of their situation. The advocate can represent the child at the discharge meeting or submits the child's comments as a report so that the whole professional system hears the child's point of view. Sometimes the child's needs and those of the parents may be at odds, and this dilemma needs to be identified and addressed by everyone involved.

> The advocate meets with Arthur during the last week of his stay. She has brought a selection of maps for Arthur to look at and she suggests they draw a map together of a treasure island. She encourages Arthur to put all his good experiences of the Croft on the island and anything he hasn't liked in the sea with the sharks. Arthur really enjoys doing this and spends a long time drawing and writing. In the centre of the island he draws musical instruments to represent the music group and in the sea he puts school.
>
> Afterwards the advocate suggests that Arthur draws his ideal island where everything is how he would like it to be. Arthur draws himself and his family on the island and a large heap of chocolate! The advocate suggests that he draws a school that he would like to go to – initially he says he wouldn't want to go to school at all, but after a discussion about the fact that he wants to be a scientist and that he will need to get some qualifications, he agrees to the task. He draws a school with lots of maps on the wall, saying that the children do 'lots of drawing and experiments and not much writing'. He also says he want there to be just a few children and nice teachers who 'smile and don't shout if your handwriting is a bit messy'.
>
> When this picture is shown in the discharge meeting it stimulates a lively discussion about Arthur's schooling and brings a sense of Arthur's personality into the room.

Creating a new story

As part of the assessment at the unit the team aim to create a coherent and detailed assessment of the child and his family that helps everyone to understand the nature of the difficulties they are facing and to construct a helpful plan. This can be boiled down to a short couple of paragraphs called a formulation. The formulation is a summary of the important factors in the child and family presentation, including risk and protective factors. This should lead to a working hypothesis that will inform the ongoing care plan for the child and family.

When David's mum, Sarah, was first seen in the outpatients department, she was at the end of her tether. Despite being well educated and articulate, her story came out in an incoherent way. She was overwhelmed by David's behaviour which had become increasingly dangerous and her unvoiced fear at that stage was that he would need to go into residential care. The voices he reported hearing reminded Sarah of her maternal aunt who had been diagnosed with schizophrenia and spent much of her life in a mental hospital. Sarah's own mental health was suffering and she blamed herself constantly for the abuse David had suffered at the hands of her ex-husband. During the admission she also admitted that, despite being close to her own mother, she felt that her mother blamed her for David's problems. David's own close relationship with his grandma reinforced Sarah's own feelings of inadequacy as a parent.

As the admission progressed Sarah gained confidence in her own parenting and this growing confidence allowed her to be more open with staff about her own depressive feelings. Some of the family therapy sessions helped to draw some clearer boundaries around her relationship with her own mother. This allowed her to see herself and her current husband as the parents who had control, whilst at the same time continuing to acknowledge the invaluable support her mother was able to give her.

David himself had been able to do some foundation work around his anxiety and his anger.

In addition much of the work at the Croft focused on giving Sarah new strategies to deal with David's very challenging behaviour and helping her co-parent with David's stepfather.

The post-traumatic stress disorder (PTSD) diagnosis was looked at carefully and it was decided that David did have some features consistent with the diagnosis, alongside other more generalised anxiety symptoms and signs of insecure attachment. It was clear that future interventions would need to bear in mind his earlier abusive history.

Story stem assessment and feedback from the observations of the team provided Sarah with some reassurance about her underlying relationship with David and highlighted how positively he felt about her. Being reassured that David was not developing a serious psychotic mental illness was also a great relief to Sarah and allowed her to think about other issues in his life. Through further discussions and observations it became very clear how attuned David was to Sarah's emotional state and how deeply affected he had been by his father's violence. It was agreed that David would need ongoing support to help him to feel more secure about relationships with adults and to reduce his worry about his mum's safety.

The formulation acknowledged that David's own anxious temperament may have been a contributory factor but that there were also significant protective factors which had emerged during the admission. These included Sarah's own willingness and emotional resources to be able to reflect and change both her attitudes and behaviours towards David and also the considerable emotional support she was receiving from her friends and her own mother.

Sarah left the Croft with increased awareness of David's emotional needs and that she would need further professional help to meet those needs. And for the first time in a very long while her own emotional needs were recognised, and a referral to adult mental health services was under way to address her own anxiety symptoms and depression.

David's school had previously perceived Sarah's own explanations as mere excuses for David's bad behaviour. They had worried that she was lacking parenting skills and were unaware of her own traumatic history.

The headteacher from the school was able to attend the discharge meeting and despite having had some initial scepticism about the admission, he was grateful for the unit teacher's practical advice regarding how to deal with David in the classroom. The school also began to appreciate some of the background factors that had contributed to David's behavioural difficulties.

The care co-ordinator from the local child mental health team was pleased to hear how much calmer Sarah felt about her son. She said that now that everyone could stop worrying about a psychotic illness the team could focus on helping David understand his anxiety and gain a sense of mastery over it. The psychologist in the community team had already spoken to her counterpart on the unit team and they had discussed an ongoing plan for David's treatment after discharge. The unit liaison nurse had made an appointment to visit Sarah and David the following week and said she would be a point of contact for the family in the weeks that followed.

Sarah's story had changed from one of 'I have a son who's sick and increasingly likely to become crazy and it's all my own fault. I'm not a fit parent' to a more measured 'Yes I did make a mistake with my marriage, but at the time I could not have known how abusive he'd turn out to be. David will not inevitably become "mad" or follow in his father's footsteps and become abusive. Yes, David's experiences have contributed to his emotional and behavioural disturbance, but with help and confidence in my own abilities this should improve over the next few years.'

David hadn't been able to articulate his own beliefs but it seemed that his story was 'Mum can't control me, I'm beyond help – I'm a bad person and will turn out like my dad.' It is hoped that his stay on the unit had helped him to begin to think, 'I'm not so bad – I'm one of the best at drawing and the teacher said I'd written one of the most imaginative stories she'd ever read. I'm very good at football and maybe I get that from my dad. I still get angry but I'm getting better at noticing it and have managed to stop myself three times here in the last week from hitting Mum! I feel much less worried about Mum – she's also going to be helped through talking to nurses and Granny can also help her.'

The role of a diagnosis or label

One of the tasks for the psychiatrists on the team is to consider whether a child might be appropriately described as having a particular mental health diagnosis as described in the classificatory systems of DSM-IV (Diagnostic and Statistical Manual of Mental Disorders) (American Psychiatric Association 1994) or ICD-10 (International Classification of Mental and Behavioural Disorders) (WHO 1992). These are manuals issued by international health organisations to describe and define diseases. The aim is to help doctors around the world to be consistent in their diagnostic approach.

There is much debate and controversy about the use and abuse of mental health labels for children and adults alike, but in the area of childhood mental health disorder the issue of labelling a child with a disorder and the implications of that process are very emotive, and often parents and professionals can have very strong views about the benefits and disadvantages of the use of such labels.

Parents may have a vested interest in their child receiving a medical diagnosis or may resist the labelling of their child. A diagnosis can be seen as a validation of the child's difficulties and as locating the difficulties in the child. Often parents say that if they don't receive a clear diagnosis for their child they feel blamed by family, neighbours, teachers and other professionals for their child's difficulties. On the other hand, some families worry that if their child is labelled they will be stigmatised and socially disadvantaged. A diagnosis can also provide access to support services, benefits, specialist education and so on and, whilst ideally resources would be allocated on the basis of a child's needs, realistically services sometimes do use diagnostic labels as a means of indexing need and rationing treatment.

A medical diagnosis can also be useful in terms of placing a child within a group of similar children, thus allowing application of knowledge from research or experience that will inform treatment or support. So, for example, if a child receives a diagnosis of Hyperkinesis syndrome (a severe form of attention deficit hyperactivity disorder), the evidence base suggests that children will benefit from stimulant medication, behaviour modification techniques and educational support (NICE 2009).

In clinical practice many children cannot be easily placed into diagnostic groups and children using tertiary services present with complex difficulties and have often had a variety of diagnoses suggested or rejected. This leaves parents, children and professionals confused and frustrated. It is a basic human trait to desire clarity and whilst in some areas of health care this can be achieved – either a bone is fractured or it is not – in the area of mental health disorders it is much harder to be dichotomous.

Most of the conditions that the team deal with have spectrums of symptomatology where the overlap between 'normal' human behaviour and 'abnormal' disorder is substantial. For example, autism is a neuro-developmental disorder, which has a strong genetic component. But rather than being inherited as a single gene condition, where the presence of one abnormal gene invariably leads to the disorder, autism is a multi-gene condition – due to this genetic variability the condition can also present in many forms and the genetic substrate is also likely to interact with various environmental influences that cause further variability in its expression in an individual. It is likely that there are individuals who have a handful of these genes in the 'normal' population who will show subtle traits of the condition but would not meet clinical criteria for the full syndrome. In autism this has been described as the 'broader phenotype' and this term has been applied to the relatives of people with autism who show subtle traits of the syndrome that may well be caused by one or more of the contributory genes present in the family (Bolton *et al.* 1994).

The situation for children with neuro-developmental conditions is further confused by the overlap between a number of developmental conditions, so children with autism can also have co-occurring conditions such as ADHD, specific learning disabilities (dyslexia), motor co-ordination disorder (dyspraxia) and a number of other difficulties.

So the application of diagnostic labels to children with multifactorial difficulties is challenging and should be undertaken with an awareness of the limitations of classificatory systems when applied to the complexity of the developing human brain.

Inherent developmental problems and care-giving styles

In trying to put together a coherent formulation or account of a child's difficulties, mental health teams look for the inherent, largely genetically determined factors that influence the child's temperament, personality and style of interacting with the world. Alongside this they consider the impact of the environment that the child is brought up in, as this also shapes the developing brain and influences the child's behaviour and emotional state. There is also the transactional nature of the relationship between the child's genetic predisposition and the care they elicit from their parents and the responses that parents elicit from their children through their parenting style.

This is a sensitive area for parents of children with special needs – like any parent they often feel responsible for all of their children's difficulties, even ones that may be biologically determined and outside their zone of influence – and the vast majority of parents are doing their utmost to ensure that their children are well cared for. As parents go through an intensive programme they will, it is hoped, acquire a clearer view of their children's strengths and difficulties and appreciate how much their style of interacting with their child can improve their child's functioning. Implicit in this last statement is that parents' interactions with their children could also cause the child to be functioning less well.

So, for example, recent research (Hughes and Ensor 2006) has shown that young children with challenging antisocial behaviour often also have poor emotional literacy and social skills – if they also live in families with high levels of criticism and a coercive style of parenting, their behavioural difficulties are much more severe than if their parents have a more nurturing and less critical approach. The message for parents is that whilst they are not the sole cause of their child's problems, how they manage the child's difficulties makes an important difference to his functioning and future outlook. This approach, sometimes known as the transactional approach, considers very closely the way children influence their environment (parents, family, peers, etc.) as well as how their environment is influencing them.

Looking at situations in a multi-factorial and holistic light is an important issue to discuss with the multi-agency network. When working with very disturbed and disturbing children it is all too easy for professionals to become very polarised themselves, thinking either that the child would be all right if only the parents were different, or that all the problems are due to the child and that the parents are the victims of their child's difficulties. If this simplistic view is not challenged then professionals may unrealistically expect that all the difficulties will be resolved if the child is placed away from his family.

How can we continue to promote change?

Once families have completed an intensive programme the question arises of how to maintain gains that have been made in a highly supported environment when families return to their home communities and a much lower level of support.

Research into human behaviour suggests that many factors influence change and some of these relate to interpersonal relationships. People are more likely to change their behaviour when they respect those advising change and see them as expert, when they feel the problem has been accurately understood and when they feel that the advisor wants the same outcome that they want. The presence of others who are following the same course of action makes change more likely, as does the perception that the change will be beneficial and that no change will be harmful.

Research into the effectiveness of treatment in children's inpatient mental health units has identified a number of factors which influence outcomes (Green and Jacobs 2004): positive treatment benefits are associated with a positive engagement of the child and parents with staff and also with the length of treatment. So whilst engagement at the outset of treatment forms the foundation for change, maintaining contact and consolidating change in the latter stages of treatment is also vital. In the setting of the Croft this translates to outpatient or outreach sessions over a period of three to six months after discharge. These sessions can take a number of forms depending on the needs of the child and family. They may be family therapy sessions, individual psychotherapy, creative therapy sessions or behaviour management support. These contacts can also encompass liaison meetings with the child's school or other agencies that will be providing ongoing support.

Family therapy

During their stay all families have family therapy sessions to aid an understanding of family functioning and to offer families a forum to consider their family history and relationships. Often it can take several weeks for the ideas in these sessions to become coherent and convergent and for some families the opportunity to continue these conversations is very valuable. The few exceptions are those for whom family therapy seemed unhelpful and those who are happier returning to their local services.

There are a number of reasons why family therapy can be useful after parents and children have left the unit.

Keeping connected

As has been mentioned earlier, many children and parents form a strong attachment to the staff, culture and building of the Croft during their very intense experience as an inpatient. Maintaining this link, in a limited form, represents both nurture and change and can reduce the sense of abandonment and loss that many families feel on departure. It allows them to create an ending over which they have more control and one which is not solely dictated by the professionals. This gradual process mirrors, in a small way, how young people leave home successfully, gradually and with regular brief contact with 'home'.

> Arthur's admission had been extended due to the slow appearance of his behavioural problems. His parents had also taken time to divulge some of his difficulties such as his bedtime problems that had initially paled into insignificance compared with some of his other behaviours. Arthur's father had also only recently been able to talk about some of his fears and concerns. It was felt by the team that the family were just starting to engage with psychological thinking at the time of Arthur's discharge.
>
> At his discharge meeting it was agreed that weekly visits by the team's liaison nurse would be offered. Her task was to support Arthur's mum in continuing with the behavioural programme around bedtime. She also made a time to see Arthur at his school and meet with his teachers. It was a great relief to Arthur's parents that they knew they were able to see a familiar member of the team after leaving. This enabled them to report how the various strategies that they had tried at the Croft were transferring to home, now that Arthur was aware he wasn't returning to the Croft on Monday mornings. As he was also just beginning to re-integrate into his local specialist education unit, it was helpful to have continuity between the approach at the unit and the approach in his new school.
>
> Arthur's parents were reassured that strategies that had been helpful during his admission would be communicated to the school. This helped them feel more confident that he would make the transfer successfully. As a child with autism, everyone was aware of his difficulties with any changes or transition and the importance of maintaining links during this phase was crucial.

Consolidating change

A six-week admission to a unit is a huge intervention in the life of a family. By definition, the majority of families who attend have been living with a child with serious difficulties that have been a major challenge to both the family and the professionals. As one referring psychiatrist put it: 'I can't expect miracles [from the unit] but you can perturb a family in a way that we can't in an outpatient setting.'

A pattern often emerges during the average six-week stay which fits with the five stages of group work process defined by Tuckman (1965): forming, norming, storming, performing and mourning. Many families experience anxiety as they settle into the Croft environment and form relationships with other parents, children and staff. They have to adjust to being exposed to a unique combination of observation and scrutiny whilst also being supported and nurtured. This process of adjustment will involve aspects of the norming, forming and performing referred to above.

It is common, after they have settled in, for families to express their anxiety by challenging behaviour towards the staff team, often accompanied by doubts about whether change will occur during the admission. This could be seen as the stage of 'storming'.

Both families and staff frequently notice change occurring as they approach the last two weeks of their stay. Parents often report change with a sense of relief and hope for the future which is then tarnished by the fear that all the progress will be lost as soon as they return home. This could be seen as the stage of 'performing', rapidly followed by 'ending' (mourning).

For some families the fear of losing the momentum for change is palpable. This is the context in which many request follow-up sessions. There is also often the reward of reuniting with 'favourite' staff members when they return to the unit.

Family therapy tries to engage the whole family, including non-resident parents or other relatives such as grandparents, and some families use these follow-on sessions to engage with family members who may have felt marginalised prior to the admission or who are holding on to the 'old' view of the child.

Using creative therapies to support change

The music therapists at the Croft also offer a service following discharge and some of these families have parallel music and family therapy sessions. Music therapy is a particularly good complement to family therapy when it is working with a particular pairing in the family. For example, when the music therapy is provided for a parent and child who have had a troubled relationship, the aim of the therapy is to enhance the parent–child relationship. Reinforcing this dyad through music therapy often consolidates earlier work started during the inpatient phase.

> After Nick and Stacey were discharged from the unit, it was decided to offer the family four monthly outpatient family therapy sessions which would include Nick, his two younger brothers, his stepfather and his mother. During the admission, Nick had initially refused to attend family therapy sessions, although his mother and stepfather had found the sessions useful to explore their own feelings regarding parenting and being parented. However, as Nick's confidence and trust had improved he had agreed to attend a family therapy session during his last week on the unit. During this session Nick had appeared to be more able than previously to hear his mother and his stepfather's views and he had asked why his younger brothers were not also attending the sessions. It was agreed, therefore, to schedule four sessions to support Nick and his family to listen to one another and to help Nick to gain a more trusting relationship with his mother and stepfather.
>
> Nick and Stacey had enjoyed music therapy sessions during their inpatient admission. It was thought that four further outpatient music therapy sessions held after the family therapy sessions would enable them to make music together and maintain the positive playful non-verbal interactions they had started to develop in previous sessions. It was also thought that these sessions might be an additional incentive to encourage Nick to return to the Croft.

'Holding' a family until other services are available

In the same way that the Croft school will sometimes continue to provide a place for a child after his inpatient stay whilst local provision is being arranged, so family therapy can serve the same function. Continuing family therapy at the unit maintains the therapeutic momentum until an appropriate resource is available in the family's local area. The therapy team aim to conduct joint meetings with the family professionals from the referring team whenever possible so that important or sensitive information can be handed over face to face. These joint meetings prevent families having to 'start from scratch' with another team, instead allowing the therapeutic conversation to continue, albeit with new therapists.

Some families feel that they have had sufficient therapeutic input at the end of their follow-up sessions and often it can be helpful for families to have a period of time without sessions to 'be ordinary' and to try out the ideas they have been talking about.

> At Patrick's discharge meeting it became clear that although the team had gone some way in understanding his difficulties, it was acknowledged that his problems were very complex and deep-seated and that despite the changes noted during his admission, his needs were still very high. Diane had made considerable progress in engaging with her son and being mindful of his needs but she had still needed the staff to help her contain Patrick's emotional lability and oppositional behaviour. The considered opinion of the multi-disciplinary team was that Patrick needed a very high level of containment and support, and they suggested that he should be considered for a therapeutic school placement.
>
> Despite the grave concerns the team had about Patrick's future, it was recognised that Diane had begun, in the last week or so, to relate to the family therapy team and to open up in ways she hadn't before. It was felt that if Patrick's family was abruptly discharged Patrick would feel uncontained and likely to return to his very risky behaviours. For this reason it was agreed that the family therapy team would offer a number of follow-up sessions in order to keep Patrick and his mum linked or 'held'. During this period they also had appointments with their local child and adult mental health (CAMH) service, and the unit liaison nurse met with family support workers who were getting to know Patrick to discuss helpful ways to gain his trust. Meanwhile Patrick's social worker used the report from the unit team to start to work with the education department to look for an appropriate placement for Patrick.

When planning transition or follow-up work with families it is important to set a clear end date if at all possible. It is all too easy for the sessions to drift and if the local service is lacking resources then the unit may be filling in a gap in their service by default.

Summary

Creating a meaningful, valid and positive story can help families to feel more confident in managing their difficulties and to be more aware of their strengths. An accurate and clear diagnosis, or acknowledgement of the complexity of their child's difficulties, will help to create consensus between families and helping agencies.

In all therapeutic settings, helping clients to transfer and maintain gains post-intervention is a challenging task. For families using intensive services, the move from high levels of specialist support back to community services can be a very anxiety-provoking one. Transitional, step-down support can ease this period and help the family to adjust and begin to live their 'new' lives.

Chapter 11

Reflection and Evolution

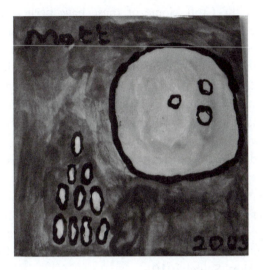

*Matt decided to do his tile on bowling, which
was his last outing at the Croft*

Introduction

Like any other health service provision, inpatient child and family
psychiatric units need to be audited and to demonstrate their quality
and effectiveness. However, as in other branches of mental health, it
is a complex task to measure outcomes in child and family psychiatry.
Each child's difficulties are so varied, treatments are individualised and
some important outcomes may rest on changes from outside the health
system. Having said this, it is important for services to get feedback
on their performance so that they can describe the outcomes for their
client group, develop their practice and benchmark themselves against
other services.

In this chapter, three different types of evaluation that have taken
place at the Croft are considered: research and audits that occur within

the unit, national audits and benchmarking, and direct feedback from children and parents.

Research and audits

Over the years there have been many research and audit projects carried out at the Croft. Some of these have been carried out by permanent staff and others by visiting trainees and students. These have all added to the knowledge base in the discipline and in turn contributed to the evolution of the service. They have included two PhD research investigations, one of which compared the newly developed music therapy diagnostic assessments (MTDAs) with established assessments of autism (Oldfield 2004). The other was concerned with a psychodynamic understanding of how autistic children understood emotions, entitled: 'Living on the edge of possibility: A study of autistic object relations' (Franke 2006). Two other studies that were of particular interest were: an investigation into whether parents' attributions, depression levels and parenting levels change during a stay at a child inpatient assessment unit (Daly and Polichroniadis 2004), and an audit of children's sleep patterns during admission (Spigel 2010).

The Croft's own patient satisfaction questionnaires have also provided some interesting results (Barker, Kenny and Wilson 2007). As might be expected, the responses were varied; however, over two-thirds of parents felt the Croft had made a difference in a positive way to their lives. Parental feedback indicated that parents particularly valued meeting other parents, and found staff very helpful and approachable. Understandably a number of parents commented on how uncomfortable it felt to be observed with their children.

A follow-up study of a group of children who attended the Croft school showed that a year later, all of them had a permanent school placement and the majority were attending school full time. Standardised measures of children's academic levels on admission and discharge to the unit school also showed significant gains in attainments during the children's admission.

These small-scale quantitative studies can provide some indicative information about the performance of the service but they do not capture the richness and depth of patients' experiences as qualitative studies might do. The direct accounts by parents and children of their experience recorded at the end of this chapter throw more light on the important processes of change taking place.

National audits and benchmarking

The Croft is an active member of the Quality Network for Inpatient Child and Adolescent Mental Health Services (QNIC), set up by the Royal College of Psychiatrists in the UK. The aim of QNIC is to provide a peer review system so that units can benchmark themselves, to improve communication between units and provide a single channel for the effective dissemination of important information from central sources such as national and professional bodies and to co-ordinate information sharing between units regarding, for example, best practice (Solomon 2009). This process follows a clinical audit cycle with self-review and peer review. In the recent QNIC review (Solomon 2009, p.8) it was noted that: 'the Croft Child and Family Unit is performing well against the QNIC service standards for another year running, showing improvements in some sections, especially Information, Consent and Confidentiality where the unit is meeting all the specified criteria'.

The Croft was also involved in an in-depth study of eight child and adolescent inpatient units commissioned by the Department of Health (Green and Jacobs 2004). The aims of this study were to look at:

- the clinical pathways leading to admission and subsequent discharge

- the change in health needs during the admission

- predictors of health gain and direct and indirect economic costs to health, social and educational services during and after treatment.

This study demonstrated the significant health gains for children and young people in all of the units studied. It found positive associations between the length of treatment, positive therapeutic alliances between child and staff, pre-admission family functioning and treatment outcome.

Children and parents' feedback

Over the years, children have talked about their experiences at the unit in a variety of ways. The section on advocacy in Chapter 10 describes one way in which children's views are heard and acknowledged. Another means of communication is through creative arts, and the pictures of the tiles at the beginning of several chapters in this book, created by children at the end of their stay at the Croft, express the experiences of their admission artistically, rather than through words.

Some children are able to express their thoughts in writing, however, and here are a few thoughts that three different children wrote about the Croft:

> *R (aged 7)*: 'I like the soft room because I like playing with the red ball. I like the badges in school when I'm good. I have lots of friends. I like playing outside and in the art room.'

> *K (aged 9)*: 'The Croft is a bit scary at first but then you get used to it and get to like it. I like the badger in the kitchen [sink disposal unit], it's amusing because it makes a funny noise. I think the soft room is a great place to play and is good when I am angry. They put you in the soft room when you are naughty or frustrated. The art room is the best place to create and make stuff like moulding clay, robots, play-dough and plasticine. The outside playground is the best place because there is a sandpit, a climbing frame, a pair of swings, a basketball net and a football goal.'

> *T (aged 12)*: T was at the Croft for four months to address insecure attachment issues and behaviour problems with her mother. During some of their admission these difficulties were tackled by helping T to become more independent and to cope with being separated from her mother.

> 'When I first came here I was scared. I really wasn't keen on coming. The staff were very welcoming and they made me feel less scared. One of my good things about the Croft is the art room because I like to make Hama beads. I like the soft room when I get to play with the shapes and the big red ball. I like school because it's not as long as normal school. At the end of the week if you've been good and earned all your stickers you can earn a badge. The stickers can

be any colour – the teacher draws cats, dogs or smiley faces. The music room is one of my favourite rooms because I love to rock out loud on the drum kit and play loads of tunes on the piano and organ. My least favourite place is the soft room when you are angry because I don't like it when you have to stay in there, it's quite frightening. I don't like the back garden when the door shuts. It locks itself and you can't get back in.

'It's very different because I have to stay at the Croft on my own. Sometimes it's just days but most of the times it's a whole week. I find it very lonely and I find it very hard to sleep because I've never been so far away from my mum before. I get to ring my mum every night at half past eight. I think that staff take good care of me when I'm on my own. The staff play games with me. Sometimes when I play outside with the staff they push me on the swings. The staff are really nice. When you are good sometimes they will walk with you to Tesco and if your mum gives you money you can spend it. When I'm on my own I have to be supervised wherever I go. There are night staff that come in the evening at nine and it depends on how old you are what time you go to bed. If you are 12 years old you're allowed to stay up to nine o'clock.'

In the final section of this chapter, two mothers of children who attended the Croft write about their experience. The two accounts are very different. At the time of writing both families were no longer inpatients or day-patients at the Croft. Veronica writes long after she and her son had been discharged but Debbie had only recently finished her stay and she and her daughter were still attending weekly outpatient music therapy sessions as well as monthly family therapy sessions. Debbie's daughter, B, had very complex needs and the Croft team felt that she had aspects of a number of different neuro-developmental and emotional disorders. Veronica's son, M, already had an established diagnosis when he came to the unit but the family were in a crisis situation that was worsening day by day.

Veronica's story is very positive and she talks generally about her admission and her son's progress. Debbie is still struggling with her daughter, and writes only about her daughter in general and about her ongoing experience as an outpatient in music therapy. Although she doesn't write directly about her inpatient stay at the Croft, the team felt that Debbie was disappointed that her daughter's difficulties had not been resolved. However, it was encouraging that she was still willing to attend outpatient sessions at the Croft and was able to make further progress within the music therapy sessions.

Debbie's story

I had B when I was 40 years old. She wasn't planned but I considered her to be a very welcome gift from God. B was an extremely quiet baby. Even though there was a lot of very noisy building going on B didn't flinch. It never upset her. She would sleep most of the time, when she was awake she didn't cry; even during the night she wouldn't cry when she was hungry, she would just stir.

Everyone including myself considered I was very lucky to have such a good baby. However, looking back now, I think there was something wrong. She was too quiet and disinterested. Although she didn't mind being picked up, she didn't seem to care either way.

B's first words were not the typical 'mamma' or 'dada', but 'Row row row' – as in the song: 'Row row row the boat'. At the same time as saying the word, she would move her upper body back and forth. This went on for a couple of months and then she just stopped speaking altogether for a very long time. At the time I remember wondering whether she would ever talk. B started to walk when she was 16 months old. She was and remains quite clumsy.

B has been looked after quite a lot by her Auntie C (my older sister) as I work full time. Both C and I noticed a dramatic change in B when she was about 20 months old. Up until this time B had been a quiet, placid child, and then one afternoon we were at home and she just seemed to open her mouth and scream for absolutely no reason. I tried everything to pacify her, she wasn't hungry, thirsty, wet or dirty. I tried playing, singing and rocking her but to no avail; this scream went on for about an hour and stopped as suddenly as it started. From then on we had a very angry, spiteful, defiant little girl, whose face would contort. She seemed to be tormented.

At present life with B is a constant battle. When B first wakes up in the morning she is like any typical six-year-old, and then after a couple of minutes a different little girl emerges. She becomes argumentative, defiant and can be aggressive. She can be a danger to herself and will think nothing of trying to touch a hot iron, cooker or kettle. She is very impulsive and will just run off into a road or anywhere the fancy takes her. B makes noises on and off throughout the day, which include throat clearing, raspberry blowing, howling like a wolf or hissing like a cat and these sounds are sometimes linked to her moving her upper body quickly back and forth. These noises occur not only at times when she is angry, they can happen if she is sitting quietly and the noises are then very quiet.

B seems to need very little sleep and will still be awake very late at night. She also will often not sleep in her own room and insists on sleeping with us in our bed. I struggle to think of a strength for B. If her determination and tenacity could be channelled into something positive then that would certainly be one of her strengths. What I enjoy about B is on the very odd occasion when you can sit with her and have a conversation far beyond her years. At these times she is like a little wise old woman and says things that are quite profound, so much so that you ask yourself: 'Where on earth did that come from?'

Before I came to the Croft I had never heard of music therapy so would never have considered it. I like to listen to music at home and B loves Michael Jackson and seems very happy when she has his DVDs on, sometimes repeating the songs over and over again. However, I didn't really see what the relevance of music therapy might be, particularly as I felt self-conscious and didn't think I had a musical bone in my body.

At first I didn't like being in the sessions with B, partly because I didn't want to be anywhere with B. However, I soon realised that the music therapist was fully aware of our circumstances and would not be judging us. It became clear that if things got out of hand the music therapist would actually be able to control the situation better than I could, so in effect I wasn't alone.

B has definitely benefited from the sessions; she is now able to tolerate not being in control all of the time. She will allow someone to sing quietly for a brief amount of time and also she has learnt (sometimes!) to say: 'stop please' instead of screaming. At times she seems to like turn-taking and sharing her music with us. I have particularly enjoyed the small pockets of co-operation I've seen in B in the music room.

I have been surprised at how much I enjoy playing the drum kit myself, and doing silly things like making little teddy bears jump up and down on the surface of the drum.

The sessions have given us a chance to do something together without all of life's difficulties getting in the way. There are moments when there is a connection and even though it might be fleeting it's a very positive thing.

Veronica's story: being a parent in the Croft

The suggestion of us attending the Croft came about at a multi-agency meeting in the April, suggested by M's psychiatrist. As parents we had reached desperation point. Life at home with our son had become intolerable. He was nine years old, accessing no education, had no self-esteem, wanted to control everything. His behaviour was violent towards us and was becoming more and more risky in general. It had resulted in a dreadful situation occurring with the police, which left him with post-traumatic stress disorder symptoms and his siblings and ourselves in emotional tatters.

We felt we were losing the battle to keep him safe and none of the statutory agencies could agree about what to do next. At the meeting it was agreed that M needed assessing holistically. This was something that had not ever happened before. There were also question marks over his diagnosis that at the time was Asperger's syndrome and ADHD (attention deficit hyperactivity disorder).

Initially we were very reluctant to go, I was under the impression it was for people who were struggling with parenting and I felt that what we needed was help with understanding what was going on for our son and also to help him. We already had three children and often in the past we had felt that we were being judged as responsible for our son's poor behaviour. It was only the thought that our other kids were managing OK that reassured us that maybe that assumption was false.

Our initial appointment to have a look around the Croft happened in the May a couple of weeks later. At that point we were at a very low ebb, we felt that we had to take this chance as there was nothing else on offer. M came with us on the visit and was very anxious and refusing to co-operate but did manage a brief game with a member of staff. We agreed that we would start at the Croft in the June. My husband and I agreed that I would attend with M and he would come up and visit as much as he could with our other children.

The night before we were due to come I was filled with mixed emotions, I felt miserable at the thought of having to stay away from home. I was terrified that it wouldn't work and we would be sent home with no one to help us at all. Equally I felt that maybe we could make some progress and at least whilst we were there I would be having the support of the staff and not having to cope at home on my own. Also it meant that his siblings could have a break from him and regain a sense of peace at home.

That first Monday morning I was really frightened as I really did not know what to expect. M was very angry about having to come and we fully expected him to run off as soon as we stopped the car. We did manage to get him inside and were met by a member of staff and shown around. The first day we spent settling in and finding out where everything was. M was actually reasonably well-behaved. We had various bits of paperwork to fill in and a meeting with staff to determine what we wanted from the Croft and a brief outline of what would be happening. While M and his dad were playing I went to chat with some of the other parents who were gathered in the lounge. Far from being the awful stereotyped 'bad parents' that I had in my head, the majority of them were ordinary just like us. From that first day I experienced a sense of camaraderie between the parents. They all knew how it felt to have a child with difficulties and I felt for the first time ever I didn't have to pretend things were OK.

My husband, M and I shared an evening meal and then I thought it would be best for him to leave. Suddenly it hit me that we were here to stay and I just wanted to run out with him. M was distraught that his dad was going and that made it harder. However, we soon got caught up in the evening activities, getting to know the other families and organising bedtime routines. It probably took until very late before M fell asleep. I finally collapsed in my bed exhausted and just sobbed.

From the next morning M was expected to join in with the Croft programme. I fully expected him to refuse to co-operate. In the morning whilst the children attended the school unit M had his tutor who had been working with him before we came into the Croft. However, the tutor couldn't make all of the sessions and M had started wanting to join in with the other children. Before long M was attending school for the first time in a very long time on a regular basis, and apart from the initial settling in teething troubles, he actually began to want to go and enjoy going and he began doing schoolwork. He also joined in with all the afternoon activities and suddenly I had some free time. It felt very unreal. The first week was very tough, I felt very emotional. I was very relieved to go home that first weekend and neither M nor I wanted to go back on the Monday morning. M had refused to come but did eventually get into the car. We gradually settled into life at the Croft. There were lots of difficult moments but lots of laughter and fun too. M and I worked hard at repairing our damaged relationship and we both gained a real sense of closeness during our time in there. We also came to value our family therapy sessions. At first I had been very reluctant to participate and could not imagine M wanting to be part of it. However, the first session he came into, he started off angry but for the first time ever, starting talking about himself and actively joining in. Some of the sessions were very emotionally difficult though and it was hard as there were times that I would have loved to have gone and shut myself in my bedroom at home and not have had to carry on at the Croft.

There were lots of highs and lows during our time at the Croft but gradually M became more responsive and the staff were able to unpeel the layers and find out who he was. It is a big bugbear of mine that there is a huge lack of services to support and work one to one with these complex children and often families have to reach crisis before any intervention happens. An important part of the Croft's work with M was helping him to gain a sense of identity, to raise his self-esteem and to give him information and support to deal with life. We also went through a diagnostic process and it was concluded that M didn't have ADHD but did have Asperger's. Some of the one-to-one work looked at encouraging M to tolerate other children and helping him to play with them. He took part in music therapy that he enjoyed very much.

I particularly enjoyed the contact with other parents, sharing stories and experiences and as we progressed through our time at the Croft, also celebrating the successes of the resident children and commiserating when days were not so good. It wasn't all fun though and whilst I was staying there was another parent attending as part of a social services request for a parenting assessment. She was particularly harsh with her child and that was very difficult to deal with. Fortunately this was one of the few negative things. Most of the parents were kind and keen to support each other.

As our time continued, we developed into quite a routine and got used to our stay. Older resident families left, to be replaced by new ones. Very soon it seemed our six-week stay was due to finish. M had changed such a lot that he was not the same boy that had arrived six weeks earlier. We had our discharge meeting which was attended by all the statutory agencies. The school staff had advised our SEN (special educational needs) education officer that M was ready and able to join in a small school group. It was decided that he would continue attending the school unit at the Croft as a day-patient until Christmas and after that he would be able to attend a small unit for children with autistic spectrum disorders. Initially M was a bit disappointed at having to come back to the Croft but it actually became the making of him. The staff continued to work closely on a one-to-one basis with him and focused on social skills, as well as the school staff working hard to bring his educational skills in line with his peers.

When he finally left, we were all relieved and also a bit sad. Here was a place that had become a bit of a home from home. It was the dedication and support that we received whilst at the Croft that enabled us to help 'turn our boy around'. It is no under-estimation to say that we got our life back...in fact better than that...we gained a happy and well-behaved boy and a family and a family life that we had never imagined possible. We are very much aware though that whilst the Croft became a turning point in our lives, it doesn't work for or isn't right for everybody. We are, however, very grateful that we had the chance to go there.

And now...M is still happy. He has done so well in his unit it is anticipated that he will begin mainstream schooling soon. He is a totally different child these days. He still has his difficulties associated with Asperger's but he now has ways to help himself. He is able to recognise when he feels stressed and understand it is OK to ask for help or to take a break. He knows that he can help calm himself when he feels anxious and he understands that Asperger's is part of him but it doesn't dominate him.

Summary

This chapter has touched on the challenging question of what the impact of an admission to a child and family psychiatric unit might be. It is a truism to say that outcomes are likely to be diverse and will depend on numerous factors, including the purpose of an admission and the nature of the child and family's difficulties on entering the unit. Although not addressed here, the question that is often not asked is what would be the outcome if any particular family did not attend the unit. Sometimes small changes that occur during the admission might set a family on a slightly different trajectory on discharge, which may lead to significant differences in outcome in the long term. The subtlety of such changes in human behaviour and the resultant change in outcome for an individual is immensely difficult to demonstrate in a systematic way. The testimony of two very different parents describing their own personal stories as well as comments from the children themselves illustrates the lived experience and the very real and important changes that frequently take place during an admission.

Appendix 1: Croft Rules

Do's	Don'ts
• Listen to each other	• Swearing
• Be kind	• Name calling
• Share with each other	• Running away from the unit
• Be gentle	
• Take turns	• Damaging property
• Have fun	• Rude gestures
• Keep your hands and feet to yourself	
• Be in the right place at the right time	

Appendix 2: Weekly Task

Name: . . . . Date: . . . .

My task for this week is

. . . .

. . . .

. . . .

. . . .

. . . .

. . . .

. . . .

. . . .

Appendix 3: Care Plan for Managing Difficult Behaviour

Name:	Hospital number:
Identified need: **No:** To identify and manage difficult behaviour effectively	**Aim:** To enable child to vent difficult feelings safely

Date	Nursing Action	Child and Family Action

	1. If child seeking information, remind them of Croft rules and state consequences if not complied with.
	
	2. If child in a state of refusal give them a choice to comply with request or have consequence implemented.
	
	3. If child becomes verbally aggressive offer time out in groups room/ soft room/garden. If child won't go then isolate child by removing others and raise the alarm.
	
	4. If child becomes physically aggressive either:
	  a. secure area by holding doors and continue observations through window
	  b. escort to designated time out place.
	
	5. When tension reduced in child staff to establish therapeutic rapport.
	
	6. Staff to complete an ABC chart.
		1. If child's parent finding it difficult to manage child's behaviour they are to make staff aware of this.
		
		2. Child's parent to make a decision regarding the level of support required from staff and to communicate this to them.
		
		3. Child's parent to co-operate with staff while managing difficult behaviour.
		
		4. Child's parent to communicate any concerns regarding the management of their child's behaviour.
		
		5. Child's parent (with child) to fill out an ABC chart.

1. 2. 3.	Evaluation	

Unit staff...
Parent/s...
Date...

Appendix 4: Children's Pictorial Timetable

9.00 Morning meeting	12.30 Lunch
9.15 Short play	13.00 Break
9.30 School	13.45 Group Monday – Art (13.30) Tuesday – Tuesday group Wednesday – Social skills Thursday – Recreation group (13.00)
10.45 Break	14.30 Break
11.15 School (apart from Wednesday when it is music)	15.00 Review of the day

Appendix 5: Parent Timetable

Day		Children	Parents
Mon	9.15	Morning meeting	
	9.30	Short play	Weekend feedback with case
	10.45	School	manager/key worker
	11.15	Break	
	12.30	School	2 p.m. Housekeeping meeting (Sandy
	1.00	Lunch	and Gerry, as required)
	1.45	Lunch break	After the day programme arrange
	2.30	Art	video if needed for Mellow Parenting
	3.00	Break	
	3.30	Review of the day	Family therapy sessions 4 p.m.–7 p.m, one session a week on a Monday or
	4.00	Residential time	Tuesday slot (Vince)
Tues	9.00	Morning meeting	
	9.15	Short play	
	9.30	School	Family therapy sessions 9.30 a.m.– 12 p.m. (Vince)
	10.45	Break	
	11.15	School	
	12.30	Lunch	2.00 p.m. Behaviour management
	1.00	Lunch break	group (Sandy, Colleen and Debbra)
	1.45	Tuesday group	June, Kelly and Mark
	2.30	Break	After the day programme arrange
	3.00	Review of the day	video if needed for Mellow Parenting
	3.30	Residential time	

Weds	9.00	Morning meeting	
	9.15	Short play	
	9.30	School	
	11.00	Break	11 a.m.–12 p.m. Parents' support
	11.45	Music group	group (Sharon and Sandy)
	12.30	Lunch	
	1.00	Lunch break	1.45 p.m.–2.30 p.m. Parents observe
	1.45	Social skills	children in social skills group
	2.30	Break	(Colleen, Andrew)
	3.00	Review of the	After the day programme arrange
		day	video if needed for Mellow Parenting
	3.30	Residential time	
Thurs	9.00	Morning meeting	
	9.15	Short play	
	9.30	School	11 a.m.–12 p.m. Mellow Parenting
	10.45	Break	group (Sharon, Sandy, Nina), not
	11.15	School	always running, please check
	12.30	Lunch	
	1.00	Recreation group	
	3.00	Review of the	1 p.m.–3 p.m. Recreation group
		day	(parents and staff)
	3.30	Residential time	
Fri	9.00	School	Weekly feedback with case manager/
	variable	Home time	key worker

Appendix 6: Assessment of Activities of Daily Living

Patient: Hospital Number:

SAFETY • Is the child aware of danger to him or herself? • Does the child pose a danger to him or herself?	
COMMUNICATION • Is communication age-appropriate? • What means are used to communicate? • Does the child seem to understand what is said to them?	
BREATHING • Is there a history of asthma or other breathing problems? • Does the child breath hold?	
FOOD AND DRINK • What does the child prefer to eat? • Does the child have any preferences of how, where or with what they eat? • Does the child have any food allergies?	
ELIMINATION • Can the child use the toilet without difficulty? • Is there any history of bed wetting or soiling?	
MOBILITY • Is the child able to move in an age-appropriate fashion? • Does the child have any problems with co-ordination or clumsiness? • Does the child fall over a lot?	

WASHING AND DRESSING • Is the child able to meet his or her own hygiene needs suitably for their age? • Are there any unusual habits in the way the child washes and dresses?	
COMFORT, REST AND SLEEP • Does the child sleep through the night? • What does the bedtime routine consist of?	
PLAY ACTIVITIES/SCHOOLING • What are the child's favourite toys/games? • Does the child play with other children? • How does the child manage at school?	
PAIN • Current medication • How does the child express his or her pain? • Is the child able to let people know how they feel? • What methods are used by the child/family to relieve pain? • Does the child have recurring illness or had major health problems?	
SELF-IMAGE • Does the child think they are good at certain things? What? • What does the child like to wear? • Is the child confident or shy?	
EMOTIONAL/SPIRITUAL NEEDS • How is the child consoled when distressed? • Does the child have a comforter or self-comforting methods? • Does the child have any spiritual or cultural beliefs/needs?	

Appendix 7: Croft Key Worker Book

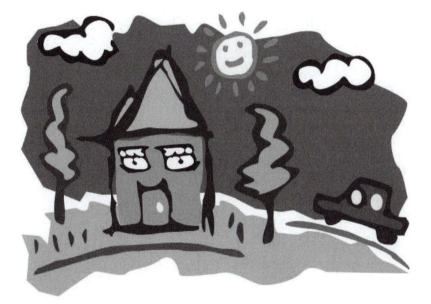

Name:

Croft Timetable

Before Programme	After Programme
1. Get washed	1. Have a snack
2. Get dressed	2. Play
3. Have breakfast	3. Have tea
4. Brush teeth	4. Quiet play
5. Line up	5. Bath
	6. Supper
	7. Cuddle time
	8. Bed

Favourite play activities:

I think I have to come to the Croft because...

- ☐ I struggle to go to school
- ☐ I am naughty
- ☐ To improve my school work
- ☐ To make friends
- ☐ The doctors need to look at the medication I am taking
- ☐ To stop fighting with my brother/sister
- ☐ I struggle to eat
- ☐ For a holiday
- ☐ To make my head better
- ☐ To give my parents a break

Any other reason:

I like doing...

1.

2.

3.

What I like and don't like eating...

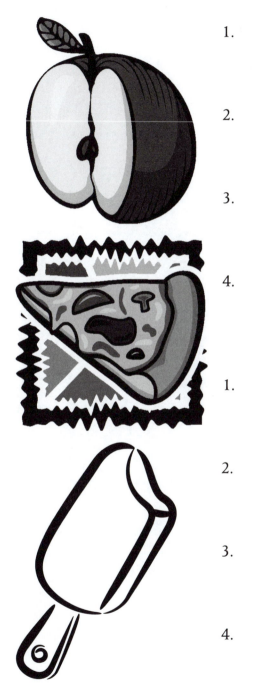

1.

2.

3.

4.

1.

2.

3.

4.

I am good at...

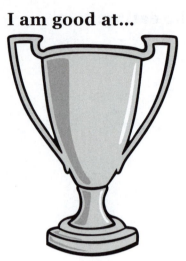

I get scared when...

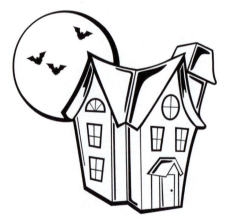

I feel happy when...

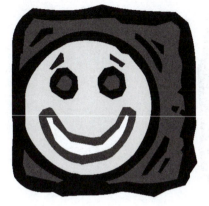

I feel sad when...

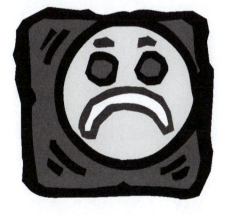

What gets me down is...

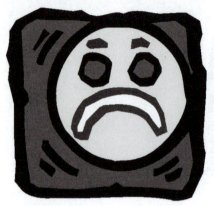

My magic moments are when...

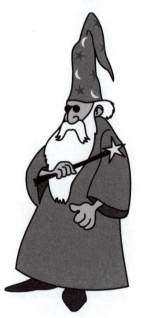

What I find difficult is...

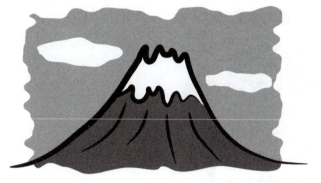

I need help when...

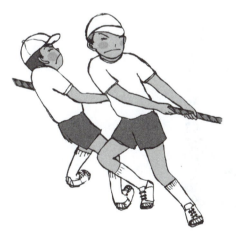

Some of my bad habits are...

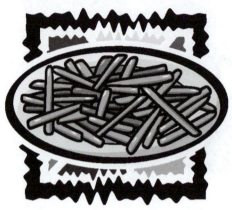

I need to work on...

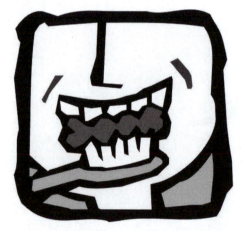

The steps I need to take are...

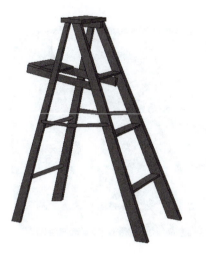

My biggest achievement is...

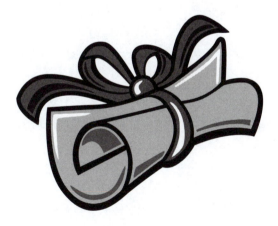

My 3 wishes are...

1.

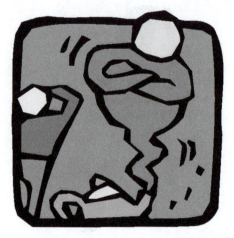

2.

3.

The good memories I will take away are...

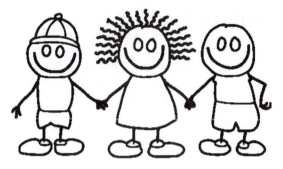

The people I need to say goodbye to are...

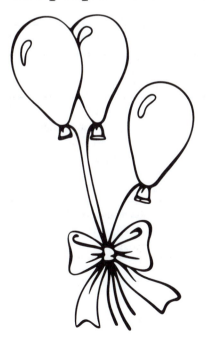

Appendix 8: Global Assessment Care Plan

Need: Diagnosis is unknown or unclear.

Aim: For a comprehensive assessment to be obtained.

Nursing action: Throughout the day staff need to observe general child behaviours as well as common signs and symptoms of several childhood disorders and record examples of these behaviours.

Signs	Examples
• impaired attention • over activity • impulsivity	• breaking off from tasks before finishing them • excessive restlessness
• defiant and provocative behaviour • persistent severe disobedience	• vandalism
• mood • excessive anxiety concerning separation • phobias	• smiling and laughing • worrying about where parents are all the time • leaving the unit
• social interactions • communication • repetitive and rigid behaviour	• lack of eye contact • how do they interpret language? • can they hold two-way interaction, e.g. conversation/play? • routines
• involuntary, rapid, re-current, non-rhythmic motor movement or vocal production	• think about situation; is it stressful? When are movements not apparent?

Source: WHO (1992) The ICD-10 Classification of Mental and Behavioural Disorders WHO

If it is noted that a child has a significant number of symptoms please implement specific care plans.

Appendix 9: Scoring of Music Therapy Diagnostic Assessment

Date:

Name of Child:

Name of Examiner:

Score in the following way: 0 = None of this behaviour was noticed

1 = Some of this behaviour was noticed

2 = A lot of this behaviour was noticed

NB: Only score if you are certain you noticed some of the behaviour. If in any doubt, do not score.

Autism spectrum disorder categories

a) Child's playing seems to be independent of therapist's playing. Therapist has to work hard to 'remain' with child and child often seems to be doing his or her own thing.

Score: . . . .

b) Child is not facially or physically engaged in playing process, or unusual eye contact (too little or too much).

Score: . . . .

c) Child doesn't make *any* spontaneous suggestions (musical or verbal) with communicative intent and/or story is excessively simple showing inability to be creative or imaginative (this should not be caused by a general learning disability, but appear untypical of the child's overall ability).

Score: . . . .

d) Child is unusually interested in structure of instruments/lines instruments or beaters up/'twiddles' with beaters or shakers/uses beaters in unexpected ways e.g. puts them in holes, sticks them on head…

Score: ………

e) Child becomes self-absorbed and difficult to distract from certain instruments such as the wind chimes or the ocean drum. (Not boredom or distractability but a more isolated, engrossed type of playing, with possible repetitive playing.)

Score: ………

f) Child's tone of voice/intonation has an unusual or repetitive quality.

Score: ………

g) Child is unable/unwilling to make up a story where we both contribute to the story line. Child may be unwilling to make up a new story rather than telling a well-known story, or child may refuse to allow the therapist to contribute in any way.

Score: ………

h) Child develops obsessive/repetitive types of playing or obsessive/repetitive patterns in story.

Score: ………

i) Child is unable to have more than one/immediate copying response. The exchanges don't develop into a dialogue.

Score: ………

j) Child is unable to have any playful or humorous exchange with the therapist.

Score: ………

k) Child wants entire session to be on his or her terms and can't accept any ideas or suggestions from the therapist. (Not in a calculated manipulative way but rather in an 'own world' way.)

Score: ………

l) Child does not show a response to therapist's singing. No embarrassment or smile or communicative response. (Do not score if child is choosing to reject or ignore the therapist and showing a negative response.)

Score: ………

Total: ………

Attention deficit disorder

a) Child has difficulties remaining engaged in any one activity for more than a few minutes.

Score: . . . .

b) Child is very distractible and fiddles with beaters or knobs on percussion instruments/child has difficulty remaining in one place/child fidgets.

Score: . . . .

Total: . . . .

Emotional/behaviour difficulties

a) Child is very anxious and/or child finds it difficult making own choices/child seems to lack a sense of self.

Score: . . . .

b) Child has difficulties moving from one activity to another/child has difficulties coming to the session or leaving the session.

Score: . . . .

c) Child seems to need to be in control of session and therapist in a 'powerful' way rather than in order to be reassured about the session.

Score: . . . .

d) Child is defiant and seems to want to draw therapist into a conflict.

Score: . . . .

e) Child is impulsive and unpredictable.

Score: . . . .

Total: . . . .

Language/learning difficulties

a) Child is difficult to understand/has pronunciation difficulties/ speaks in an ungrammatical way (more so than age of child would lead you to expect).

Score: ....

b) Child speaks very little or not at all and/or child seems very anxious about speaking. (Do not score when therapist feels child is making a point of not speaking but only if it is felt that child has real difficulties in this area.)

Score: ....

c) Child has difficulties understanding the therapist.

Score: ....

d) Child is clumsy or awkward/unco-ordinated.

Score: ....

Total: ....

Cut-off points: Autism: 10

Autism spectrum: 6

Attention deficit disorder: 3

Emotional/behaviour difficulties: 5

Language/learning difficulties: 4

References

Achenbach, T.M. and Rescorla, L.A. (2001) *Manual for the ASEBA School-Age Forms and Profiles.* Burlington, VT: University of Vermont, Research Center for Children, Youth and Families.

Ainsworth, M.D.A., Blehar, M.C., Waters, E. and Wall, S. (1978) *Patterns of Attachment: A Psychological Study of the Strange Situation.* Hillsdale, NJ: Erlbaum.

American Psychiatric Association (1994) *Diagnostic and Statistical Manual of Mental Disorders* (4th edition). Washington, DC: American Psychiatric Press.

Andersen, T. (1987) 'The reflecting team: Dialogue and meta dialogue.' *Family Process 26,* 415–428.

Anderson, V., Northam, E., Hendy, J. and Wrennall, J. (2001) *Developmental Neuropsychology: A Clinical Approach.* Hove: Psychology Press Ltd.

Asen, E. (2002) 'Multi-family therapy: An overview.' *Journal of Family Therapy 24,* 3–16.

Barker, H., Kenny, S. and Wilson, C. (2007) 'Croft annual report.' Unpublished.

Barker, J. and Modes, D. (2004) *The Child in Mind – A Child Protection Handbook.* London: Routledge.

Baron-Cohen, S. (2008) *Autism and Asperger Syndrome: The Facts.* Oxford: Oxford University Press.

Bateson, G. (1972) *Steps to an Ecology of Mind.* New York: Ballantyne.

Bernard, J.M. and Goodyear, R.K. (2004) *Fundamentals of Clinical Supervision.* London: Pearson.

Blom-Cooper, L. (1985) *A Child in Trust: Jasmine Beckford.* London: Brent.

Bolton, P., Macdonald, H., Pickles, A., Rios, P. *et al.* (1994) 'A case-control family history study of autism.' *Journal of Child Psychology and Psychiatry 35,* 5, 877–900.

Bowlby, J. (1951) *Maternal Care and Mental Health.* New York: Schocken.

Bowlby, J. (1998) *A Secure Base: Clinical Application of Attachment Theory.* London: Tavistock/ Routledge.

Bretherton, I., Oppenheim, D., Buchsbaum, H. and Emde, R. (1990) *MacArthur Story Stem Battery Coding Manual.* The MacArthur Narrative Group (unpublished).

British Psychological Society, The (2007) *Attachment Theory into Practice.* Briefing Paper no 26. Leicester: Division of Clinical Psychology, Faculty of Children and Young People.

Buchalter, S. (2009) *Art Therapy Techniques and Applications.* London: Jessica Kingsley Publishers.

Cairns, K. (2004) 'Living with Children Who Think and Feel With a Different Brain.' In R. Philips (ed.) *Children Exposed to Parental Substance Misuse* (Ch. 4). London: British Association for Adoption and Fostering.

Cameron, C.L. (2007) 'Single session and walk-in psychotherapy: A descriptive account of the literature.' *BACP Journal Counselling and Psychotherapy Research 7,* 4, 245–249.

Cantwell, D.P. (1991) 'Association between attention deficit-hyperactivity disorder and learning disorders.' *Journal of Learning Disabilities 24,* 2, 88–95.

Carr, A. (2006) *Handbook of Child and Adolescent Clinical Psychology.* London: Taylor and Francis.

Carter, B. and McGoldrick, M. (1999) *The Changing Family Life Cycle: A Framework for Family Therapy.* Boston, MA: Allyn and Bacon.

Carter, E. and Oldfield, A. (2002) 'A Music Therapy Group to Assist Clinical Diagnoses in Child and Family Psychiatry.' In A. Davies and E. Richards (eds) *Group Work in Music Therapy*. London: Jessica Kingsley Publishers.

Cassidy, J. (1994) 'Emotion regulation: Influences of attachment relationships.' *Monographs for the Society of Research in Child Development 59*, 228–249.

Cecchin, G. (1987) 'Hypothesising, circularity and neutrality revisited.' *Family Process 26*, 405–413.

Conners, C.K. (1997) *Conners Rating Scales-Revised.* Toronto, ON: Multi-Health Systems, Inc.

Cottrell, D., Fonagy, P., Kurtz, Z., Phillips, J. and Target, M. (2005) *What Works for Whom? A Critical Review of Treatments for Children and Adolescents.* London: Routledge.

Crittenden, P.M., Landini, A. and Claussen, A.H. (2001) 'A Dynamic-Maturational Approach to Treatment of Maltreated Children.' In J.N. Hughes, A.M. La Greca and J.C. Conoley (eds) *Handbook of Psychological Services for Children and Adolescents.* Oxford: Oxford University Press.

Croft, W. (2004) 'The impact on parents of being observed in a children's in-patient unit: Does it help or hinder the collaboration process and what factors influence it?' Unpublished manuscript, University of East Anglia.

Dahl, R. (1982) *The BFG.* London: Penguin Books Ltd.

Daly, J. and Polichroniadis, M. (2004) 'Do parents' attributions, depression levels and parenting stress levels change during a stay at a child in-patient assessment unit?' Unpublished research report.

Daniel, B., Wassell, S. and Gilligan, R. (1999) 'It's just common sense isn't it? Exploring ways of putting theory of resilience into actions.' *Adoption and Fostering 23*, 3, 6–15.

de Shazer, S. (1988) *Clues: Investigating Solutions in Brief Therapy.* New York: Norton.

de Shazer, S., Berg, I.K., Lipchik, E., Nunally, E. *et al.* (1986) 'Brief therapy: Focused solution development.' *Family Process 25*, 2, 207–221.

DH (Department of Health) (2000) *Working Together to Safeguard Children: A Guide to Inter-agency Working to Safeguard and Promote the Welfare of Children.* London: DH.

Drost, J. (2006) *The Bubblegum Guy: How To Deal With How You Feel.* London: Sage Publications.

Duhl, F., Kantor, D. and Duhl, B.S. (1973) 'Learning, Space and Action in Family Therapy: A Primer of Sculpture.' In D. Bloch (ed.) *Techniques of Family Psychotherapy: A Primer.* New York: Grune and Stratton.

Edgin, J.O. and Pennington, B.F. (2005) 'Spatial cognition in autistic spectrum disorders: Superior, impaired or just intact?' *Journal of Autism and Developmental Disorders 35*, 6, 729–745.

Emslie, H., Wilson, F.C., Burden, V., Nimmo-Smith, I. and Wilson, B. (2003) *Behavioural Assessment of the Dysexecutive Syndrome in Children (BADS-C).* San Antonio, TX: Pearson.

Flaskas, C. (1996) 'Understanding the Therapeutic Relationship: Using Psychodynamic Ideas in the Systemic Context.' In C. Flaskas and A. Perles (eds) *The Therapeutic Relationship in Systemic Therapy.* London: Karnac Books.

Fox, H. (2003) 'Using therapeutic documents: A review.' *The International Journal of Narrative Therapy and Community Work 3*, 26–36.

Franke, C. (2006) 'Living on the edge of possibility: A study of autistic object relations.' PhD thesis, University of Essex.

Friedberg, R.D. and McClure, J.M. (2002) *Clinical Practice of Cognitive Therapy with Children and Adolescents. The Nuts and Bolts.* New York: Guilford Press.

George, E., Iveson, C. and Ratner, H. (1990) *Problem to Solution.* London: BT Press.

Goodyer, I.M. (2001) *The Depressed Child and Adolescent* (2nd edition). Cambridge: Cambridge University Press.

Green, J. and Jacobs, B. (2004) 'Children and young persons inpatient evaluation (CHYPIE) study of the process, outcome and economics of child and adolescent psychiatry inpatient treatment.' Conference proceedings for 'Informing the Future of Inpatient CAMHS.' London.

Green, J., Jacobs, B., Beecham, J., Dunn, G., Kroll, L., Tobias, C. and Briskman, J. (2007) 'Inpatient treatment in child and adolescent psychiatry: A prospective study of health gain and costs.' *Journal of Child Psychology and Psychiatry 48*, 1259–1267.

Haigh, R. (2000) 'Support systems (2): Staff sensitivity groups.' *Advances in Psychiatric Treatment 6*, 312–319.

Hemmings, P. (2003) *All About Me Game.* London: Barnardo's.

Henggeler, S.W., Melton, G.B., Smith, L.A., Schoenwald, S.K. and Hanley, J. (1993) 'Family preservation using multisystemic treatment: Long term follow-up to a clinical trial with serious juvenile offenders.' *Journal of Child and Family Studies 2*, 283–293.

Henggeler, S.W., Schoenwald, S.K., Borduin, C.M., Rowland, M.D. and Cunningham, P.B. (2009) *Multisystemic Therapy for Antisocial Behavior in Children and Adolescents (Treatment Manuals for Practitioners).* New York: Guilford Press.

Hesketh, V. and Olney, S. (2004) 'Working with Families in a School Setting.' In J. Wearmouth, R. Richmond, T. Glynn and M. Berryman (eds) *Understanding Pupil Behaviour in Schools.* London: Open University Press.

Hodges, J., Steele, M., Hillman, S. and Henderson, K. (2003) 'Mental Representations and Defences in Severely Maltreated Children: A Story Stem Battery and Rating System for Clinical Assessment and Research Applications.' In R.N. Emde, D.P. Wolf and D. Oppenheim (eds) *Revealing the Inner Worlds of Young Children: The MacArthur Story Stem Battery and Parent-Child Narratives.* Oxford: Oxford University Press.

Holmes, J. (2002) 'Acute wards: Problems and solutions.' *Psychiatric Bulletin 26*, 383–385.

Howe, D., Brandon, M., Hinings, D. and Schofield, G. (1999) *Attachment Theory, Child Maltreatment and Family Support: A Practice Model.* New York: Palgrave.

Hughes, C. and Ensor, R. (2006) 'Behavioural Problems in Two-Year-Olds: Links with Individual Differences in Theory of Mind, Executive Function and Negative Parenting.' *Journal of Child Psychology & Psychiatry 47*, 488–497.

Humphrey, A. (2006) 'Children behaving badly – a case of misunderstanding? The development of a CAMHS based child neuropsychology service.' *The Psychologist 19*, 8, 494–495.

Hyland, P. (1990) 'Family therapy in hospital treatment of children and adolescents.' *Bulletin of the Mennenger Clinic 54*, 1, 48–63.

Jenkins, A. (1990) *Invitations to Responsibility.* Adelaide: Dulwich Centre Publications.

Kennedy, R., Heymans, A. and Tischler, L. (eds) (1987) *The Family as In-patient: Families and Adolescents.* London: Cassel Publications, West London Mental Health NHS Trust.

Kenny, S. (2001) 'The experience and meaning of close observation on an in-patient adolescent ward.' MSc Dissertation for M19 Institutional and Community Care. London: The Tavistock Centre and Middlesex University.

Kerr, C. (1999) *Calm for Kids.* Available at www.calmforkids.com, accessed on 27 January 2011.

Kerr, C. (2009) 'Children's yoga and relaxation, Module 2.' Unpublished teaching material distributed on a training course, London, June.

Lang, P. and Little, M. (1990) 'The systemic professional: Domains of action and the question of neutrality.' *Human Systems 1*, 39–55.

Legoff, D.B. and Sherman, M. (2005) 'Long-term outcome of social skills intervention based on interactive LEGO play.' *Autism 10*, 1–31.

Linehan, M.M., Dimeff, L.A. and Koerner, K. (2007) *Dialectical Behavior Therapy in Clinical Practice: Applications across Disorders and Settings.* New York: Guilford Press.

Lines, D. (2007) *The Bullies: Understanding Bullies and Bullying.* London: Jessica Kingsley Publishers.

Locke, L.M. and Prinz, R.J. (2002) 'Measurement of parental discipline and nurturance.' *Clinical Psychology Review 22*, 6, 895–929.

Laming, Lord (2003) *The Victoria Climbié Inquiry: Report of an Inquiry by Lord Laming.* London: Stationery Office.

Lord, C., Rutter, M., Goode, S., Heemsbergen, J. *et al.* (1989) 'Autism diagnostic observation schedule: A standardised observation of communicative and social behavior.' *Journal of Autism and Developmental Disorders 19*, 185–212.

Lord, C., Rutter, M. and LaCouteur, A. (1994) 'Autism diagnostic interview-revised: A revised version of a diagnostic interview for caregivers of individuals with possible pervasive developmental disorders.' *Journal of Autism and Developmental Disorders 24*, 659–685.

McFarlane, W.R., Dixon, L., Lukens, E. and Lucksted, A. (2003) 'Family psychoeducation and schizophrenia: A review of the literature.' *Journal of Marital and Family Therapy 29*, 2, 223–245, April.

Main, M. and Solomon, J. (1986) 'Discovery of an Insecure Disorganized Attachment Pattern: Procedures, Findings and Implications for Classification of Behaviour.' In M. Yogman and T.C. Brazelton (eds) *Affective Development in Infancy.* Norwood, NJ: Ablex.

Mason, B. (1993) 'Towards a position of safe uncertainty.' *Journal of Human Systems 4*, 3–4, 259–265.

Meltzer, H. and Gatward, R. with Goodman, R. and Ford, T. (2000) *The Mental Health of Children and Adolescents in Great Britain: Summary Report.* London: The Stationery Office.

Menzies Lyth, I. (1988) *Containing Anxiety in Institutions: Selected Essays* (Volume 1). London: Free Association Books.

Miller, W.R. and Rollnick, S. (2002) *Motivational Interviewing: Preparing People for Change.* London: Guilford Press.

Minuchin, S. (1974) *Families and Family Therapy.* Cambridge, MA: Harvard University Press.

Minuchin, S. and Fishman, H.C. (1981) *Family Therapy Techniques.* Cambridge, MA: Harvard University Press.

Muir, E., Lojkasek, M. and Cohen, N. (1999) *Wait, Watch and Wonder, A Manual Describing a Dynamic Infant Led Approach in Infancy and Childhood.* Toronto: The Hinks-Dellcrest Centre, Gail Appel Institute.

NHS Management Executive (1993) *A Vision for the Future. The Nursing, Midwifery and Health Visiting Contribution to Health and Health Care.* Cm. 5730. London: Department of Health.

NICE (National Institute for Health and Clinical Excellence) (2006) *Parent Training/Education Programmes in the Management of Children with Conduct Disorders.* London: NICE.

NICE (2009) *Attention Deficit Hyperactivity Disorder: Diagnosis and Management of ADHD in Children, Young People and Adults.* NICE Clinical Guideline 72. London: NICE.

Ofsted (2009) *Inspection Report: Pilgrim PRU.* Cambridge: The Darwin Centre, 17 March.

O'Herlihy, A., Worrall, A., Banerjee, S., Jaffa, T. *et. al.* (2001) 'National In-patient Child and Adolescent Psychiatry Study (NICAPS).' London: Royal College of Psychiatrists Research Unit. Available at www.rcpsych.ac.uk/quality/research/completedprojects/nicaps.aspx, accessed on 28 January 2011.

Oldfield, A. (2004) 'Music Therapy with Children on the Autistic Spectrum: Approaches Derived from Clinical Practice and Research.' PhD thesis, Anglia Ruskin University.

Oldfield, A. (2006) *Interactive Music Therapy in Child and Family Psychiatry: Clinical Practice, Research and Teaching.* London: Jessica Kingsley Publishers.

Oldfield, A. and Nudds, J. (2005) *The Croft: A Unit for Child and Family Psychiatry in Cambridge.* Training video produced by Anglia Ruskin University, available from the British Society for Music Therapy.

Palazzoli, S.M., Boscolo, L., Cecchin, G. and Prata, G. (1980a) 'Hypothesising, circularity and neutrality: Three guide lines for the conductor of a session.' *Family Process 9*, 3–12.

Palazzoli, S.M., Boscolo, L., Cecchin, G. and Prata, G. (1980b) 'The problem of the referring person.' *Journal of Marital and Family Therapy 6*, 3–9.

Parsons, C. (1998) 'Trends in exclusion from school.' *FORUM 40*, 1, 11–14.

Penn, P. (1982) 'Circular questioning.' *Family Process 21*, 267–280.

Pennington, B.F. and Ozonoff, S. (1996) 'Executive functions and developmental psychopathology.' *Journal of Child Psychology and Psychiatry 37*, 51–87.

Phelan, T. (2003) *1-2-3 Magic: Effective Discipline for Children 2–12.* Glen Ellyn, IL: Child Management Inc.

Prochaska, J.O., DiClemente, C.C. and Norcross, J.C. (1992) 'In search of how people change: Applications to addictive behaviors.' *American Psychologist 47*, 1102–1114.

Puckering, C. (2004) 'Parenting in Social and Economic Adversity.' In M. Hoghughi and N. Long (eds) *Handbook of Parenting: Theory and Research for Practice.* London: Sage Publications.

Puckering, C., Rogers, J., Mills, M., Cox, A.D. and Mattsson-Graff, M. (1994) 'Process and evaluation of a group intervention for mothers with parenting difficulties.' *Child Abuse Review 3*, 299–310.

Richer, J. and Coates, S. (eds) (2001) *Autism – The Search for Coherence.* London: Jessica Kingsley Publishers.

Rivington, L. (2008) 'Parents resident with their children at the Croft Child Psychiatric Inpatient Unit: A study of the parents' perspective of the experience.' Unpublished manuscript. Research dissertation submitted for MSc Degree in Family and Systemic Psychotherapy, Birkbeck College, University of London, in collaboration with the Institute of Family Therapy.

Rolf, H. (2001) 'Patterns of consistency and deviation in therapists' counter-transference feelings.' *Journal of Psychotherapy Research and Practice 9*, 136–141.

Rutter, M. (2006) 'Is Sure Start an effective preventive intervention?' *Child and Adolescent Mental Health 11*, 3, 135–141.

Sameroff, A.J., McDonough, S.C. and Rosenblum, K.L. (2004) *Treating Parent-Infant Relationship Problems.* New York: Guilford Press.

Schore, A.N. (2001) 'Effects of a secure attachment relationship on right brain development, affect regulation and infant mental health.' *Infant Mental Health Journal 22*, 201–269.

Shapiro, L.E. (1994) *Short-Term Therapy with Children.* Indiana, PA: Center for Applied Psychology, Indiana University of Pennsylvania.

Sinason, V. (1992) *Mental Handicap and the Human Condition.* London: Free Association Books.

Smith, J. (2008) 'Fools rush in where angels fear to tread: An exploration and reflection upon the assessment process in psychotherapy and counselling.' Thesis submitted to University of Cambridge.

Solomon, J. (ed.) (2009) *Quality Network for In-patient CAMHS (QNIC): The Croft Child and Family unit; Review Summary – Final Report, August.* London: Royal College of Psychiatrists. Unpublished report available from the Croft Children's Unit, Cambridge.

Speck, P. (1994) 'Working with Dying People: On Being Good Enough.' In A. Obholzer and V. Roberts (eds) *The Unconscious at Work.* London: Routledge.

Spigel, S. (2010) 'Recording sleep difficulties amongst children admitted to an inpatient unit.' Unpublished audit.

Stallard, P. (2002) *Think Good, Feel Good: A Cognitive Therapy Workbook for Children and Young People.* Chichester: Wiley Blackwell.

Stein, M. (2004) *What Works for Young People Leaving Care?* Ilford: Barnardo's.

Stern, D.N. (2004) 'The Motherhood Constellation.' In A.J. Sameroff, S.C. McDonough and K.L. Rosenblum (2004) *Treating Parent-Infant Relationship Problems.* New York: Guilford Press.

Tomm, K. (1987) 'Interventive interviewing, Part 1: Strategising as a fourth guideline for the therapist.' *Family Process 26,* 167–183.

Tronnick, E.Z. (1989) 'Emotions and emotional communication in infants.' *American Psychologist 44,* 2, 112–119.

Tuckman, B. (1965) 'Developmental sequence in small groups.' *Psychological Bulletin 63,* 6, 384–399.

Ward, A., Kasinski, K., Pooley, J. and Worthington, A. (2003) *Therapeutic Communities for Children and Young People.* Community, Culture and Change Series No 10. London: Jessica Kingsley Publishers.

Watzlawick, P., Weakland, J. and Fisch, R. (1974) *Change: Principles of Problem Formation and Problem Resolution.* New York: Norton.

Wechsler, D. (2003) *The Wechsler Intelligence Scale for Children* (4th edition). San Antonio, TX: Pearson.

White, M. and Epston, D. (1989) *Literate Means to Therapeutic Ends.* Adelaide: Dulwich Centre Publications.

WHO (World Heath Organization) (1992) *International Classification of Diseases, Mental and Behavioural Disorders.* Geneva: WHO.

Willicut, E.G. and Pennington, B.F. (2000) 'Psychiatric comorbidity in children and adolescents with reading disability.' *Journal of Child Psychology and Psychiatry and Allied Disciplines 41,* 1039–1048.

Winship, G. (1995) 'The unconscious impact of caring for acutely disturbed patients.' *Journal of Psychiatric and Mental Health Nursing 2,* 2, 227–233.

Yalom, I.D. (1985) *In-Patient Group Psychotherapy.* New York: Basic Books.

Yule, W., Smith, P. and Perrin, S. (2004) 'Post-Traumatic Stress Disorders.' In. P.J. Graham, *Cognitive Behaviour Therapy for Children and Families.* Cambridge: Cambridge University Press.

Zeenah, C.H. (2000) *Handbook of Infant Mental Health.* New York: Guilford Press.

Subject Index

Author Index